National Registry Paramedic Prep

Ace the National Paramedic Exam on Your First Try | Practice Questions, Detailed Answer Explanations & Test-Taking Tips to Score a 98% Pass Rate

Berwin Johnson

Copyright © 2023 Berwin Johnson

All rights reserved.

Table of Contents

Introduction

Welcome to *"National Registry Paramedic Prep"* — your ultimate guide to passing the National Registry Paramedic Exam and becoming a certified paramedic professional.

This book has been meticulously crafted to provide you with the knowledge, strategies, and tools necessary to excel in this challenging certification exam. The first section of *"National Registry Paramedic Prep"* lays the foundation for success by exploring essential test-taking tips such as overcoming test anxiety, developing an effective study strategy, and mastering time management techniques. Understanding these vital exam preparation concepts will ensure that you are well equipped for the rigorous National Registry Paramedic Exam.

Our comprehensive coverage of paramedic certification content begins with an overview of the National Registry Paramedic Exam itself. We delve into key concepts and skills assessed on the exam, providing you with all the essential information you need to succeed. Topics covered range from anatomy and physiology to pharmacology and medication administration, with special sections dedicated to airway management, patient assessment, and life span development.

In addition to thorough explanations of medical emergencies and lessons on trauma management, *"National Registry Paramedic Prep"* also includes focused chapters on specific aspects of paramedics' scope of practice including gynecology, obstetrics, and newborn resuscitation.

Moreover, this book covers essential aspects beyond medical knowledge such as EMS operations, incident command systems, medical legal considerations, ethical dilemmas in paramedicine practice, and documentation standards. To optimize your learning experience and solidify your understanding of concepts covered throughout this book, we provide comprehensive practice exams consisting of 135 multiple-choice questions. As you work through these questions, you will gain invaluable insights into areas where you may need further study or practice.

Finally, no preparation would be complete without understanding the rationale behind each answer provided. Our practice exams come with detailed explanations and supporting information that will help clarify any uncertainties or misconceptions encountered during your course of study.

Embark on your journey to becoming a certified paramedic by immersing yourself in the pages of *"National Registry Paramedic Prep."* Let this book be your trusted partner as you pursue your dream career in paramedicine.

Chapter 1

How To Pass National Registry Paramedic Exam

As a paramedic student, you have spent countless hours in the classroom, reading textbooks, and participating in clinical rotations to gain the knowledge and skills necessary for your field. Now it is time to prepare for the National Registry Paramedic Exam (NRPE), a crucial step toward obtaining your paramedic license.

In this chapter, we will provide helpful test tips for navigating the NRPE successfully. By following these guidelines, you can increase your chances of success and move closer to your goal of becoming a licensed paramedic.

1. **Familiarize yourself with the exam structure:** The NRPE consists of two parts: a cognitive (computer-based) test and a psychomotor (practical) test. The cognitive exam assesses your knowledge of paramedicine principles, while the psychomotor exam evaluates your ability to perform critical tasks in real-life scenarios. In total, the exam will contain between 80-150 questions covering various topics.

2. **Review the NREMT content outline:** The National Registry of Emergency Medical Technicians (NREMT) provides an outlined list of topics covered on the exam. Review these subject areas carefully to identify areas where you may need additional study or practice.

3. **Create a study schedule:** A consistent and well-planned study schedule is crucial to success on the NRPE. Allocate time daily to review essential materials such as textbooks, class notes, and practice exams. Give yourself enough time before exam day to cover all topic areas thoroughly.

4. **Utilize multiple study resources:** Taking advantage of diverse study resources can enhance your understanding of essential concepts and improve retention. Consider using informative textbooks, flashcards, online quizzes, video lectures, and joining study groups to encourage discussion and collaborative learning.

5. **Take practice exams:** Practice exams are an invaluable resource for assessing your readiness for the NRPE. They can help determine where you need to focus your studies and give you a sense of what to expect from the actual exam. Furthermore, timed practice exams will help you improve on time management skills.

6. **Master your test-taking strategies:** Familiarize yourself with various test-taking strategies, such as eliminating incorrect answer choices, reading questions carefully, and answering the questions you know first before moving onto more challenging ones. Practicing these techniques can be helpful in managing stress during the exam.

7. **Prepare for the psychomotor exam:** Ensure that you know each skill station's guidelines by reviewing them beforehand and practicing them at home or school. The practical portion of your NRPE is crucial to demonstrate your ability to perform essential paramedic tasks.

8. **Rest well and eat healthily:** A refreshed mind and healthy body are critical for optimal test performance. Ensure that you get plenty of sleep in the week leading up to the exam, and maintain a balanced diet.

9. **Stay organized on exam day:** Arrive early on exam day with all required documents and materials such as your photo ID, test confirmation, and up-to-date CPR card. Gather these documents well ahead of time to avoid any last-minute complications.

10. **Manage stress effectively:** Exam anxiety can hinder performance if not managed properly. Establish relaxation techniques such as deep breathing exercises, visualization, or meditation to help alleviate stress during the NRPE.

11. **Learn from your mistakes:** If you do not succeed on your initial attempt at the NRPE, don't be discouraged! Reflect on your performance and identify where improvements can be made for future attempts.

By following these test tips along with consistent effort in both your study habits and clinical practice, you will increase your chances of success in passing the National Registry Paramedic Exam. Remember that preparation is key; so, invest enough time in understanding both the theoretical concepts and practical skills essential for paramedical practice.

How To Overcome Test Anxiety

As you prepare for the National Registry Paramedic Exam, one of the most critical factors contributing to your success is the ability to manage test anxiety. Such anxiety can cause mental blocks, impair your focus, and hinder your performance on exam day. Let's discuss various strategies to help you overcome test anxiety and confidently tackle the exam.

1. **Identify the root cause of your anxiety:** To overcome test anxiety, you first need to understand why it occurs. Some common reasons include fear of failure, lack of preparation, or previous poor exam performance. Reflect on your experiences and pinpoint the source of your stress. Acknowledging the cause enables you to develop targeted strategies to cope with your anxiety.

2. **Develop a solid study plan:** A well-structured study plan can improve your confidence and alleviate test-related stress. Break down the material into smaller sections and create a schedule based on the time you have available before the exam. Ensure that you allocate enough time for each topic and include regular review sessions in your plan.

3. **Utilize effective study techniques:** Efficient study methods are key to retaining information effectively and boosting confidence during pre-exam preparation. Useful techniques include:

   – *Active reading:* Highlight important points in textbooks, take notes, and ask yourself questions as you read.

   – *Practice tests:* Take advantage of online resources offering practice exams to help familiarize yourself with question types and gauge your progress.

   – *Teaching others:* Explain topics to someone else or give a mock presentation on a subject.

4. **Focus on maintaining a healthy lifestyle:** Ensure that you prioritize self-care by following a healthy lifestyle as part of your preparation process. Proper nutrition, physical activity, and sufficient sleep all positively impact cognitive function and stress management:

   – *Nutrition:* Consume a well-balanced diet rich in fruits, vegetables, lean proteins, and whole grains to fuel your brain and body efficiently.

   – *Exercise:* Engage in a regular exercise routine to increase endorphin levels, reduce stress, and improve focus.

   – *Sleep:* Aim for 7-9 hours of sleep per night, establishing a regular sleep schedule to ensure mental alertness and optimal cognitive function.

5. **Employ relaxation techniques:** Incorporate relaxation exercises into your routine to help manage stress and reduce anxiety. Some techniques to consider include:

   – *Deep breathing exercises:* Regulate breathing patterns by focusing on taking slow, deep breaths when you feel tense or overwhelmed.

   – *Progressive muscle relaxation:* Tense each muscle group for a few seconds before releasing tension, working from head to toe.

   – *Mindfulness meditation:* Practice mindfulness by focusing on the present moment, accepting any thoughts or emotions that arise without judgment.

6. **Develop test-taking strategies:** Familiarize yourself with exam format and layout, allowing you to develop useful test-taking strategies to minimize stress on test day:

   – *Have a personalized plan:* Know what sections you need to complete first and allocate

11

time accordingly.

- *Manage your time effectively:* Maintain a steady pace during the exam, being mindful of time constraints.

- *Answer questions strategically:* Prioritize questions with which you are familiar before attempting more complex questions.

7. **Embrace a positive mindset:** Maintain an optimistic attitude throughout the preparation process, focusing on strengths and progress rather than dwelling on past mistakes. Encourage yourself through positive affirmations and visualize success on exam day. Remember that no one is perfect - accept that setbacks will occur but treat them as opportunities for growth.

8. **Seek support:** If necessary, do not hesitate to seek help from friends, family members, or school counselors for advice or support during your preparation phase. Stay active in study groups or online forums dedicated to discussing paramedic exam topics to glean insights from others' experiences.

9. **Practice stress-relief techniques on exam day:** Finally, implement stress-management techniques on the day of the exam to keep anxiety at bay:

- *Arrive early:* Allow ample time to arrive at the testing center, check-in, and acclimate to your surroundings.

- *Take regular breaks:* Pause periodically during the exam if allowed. Use breaks to stretch, practice deep breathing exercises, or recite positive affirmations.

- *Stay focused:* Refrain from comparing yourself to others or obsessing over specific questions.

Step-By-Step Study Strategy

The exam is a comprehensive assessment of your knowledge and skills in emergency medical care. To perform well on this test, you need a strategic approach to studying—one that maximizes your chances of success. This section will provide you with an effective study strategy, complete with tips and techniques geared towards managing time, optimizing resources, and enhancing recall.

Step 1: Understand the Exam Structure

Before you start studying, it is essential to familiarize yourself with the test format and content areas. The National Registry Paramedic Exam consists of two main components: the Cognitive Exam and the Psychomotor Exam. The Cognitive Exam evaluates your knowledge of emergency care through a computer-based, adaptive test consisting of 80-150 questions. On the other hand, the Psychomotor Exam assesses your abilities in carrying out critical, hands-on tasks.

Make sure you are well-versed in each content area covered by the Cognitive Exam. These include:

- Airway, Respiration & Ventilation

- Cardiology & Resuscitation
- Trauma
- Medical & Obstetrics/Gynecology
- EMS Operations

Having a solid understanding of these domains will give you an edge in tackling challenging questions head-on.

Step 2: Set Clear Goals & Plan Your Study Session

Next, establish measurable objectives and timeframe for your preparation. Are there specific topics you need to focus on? How many hours per week do you plan on dedicating to studying? Break down your goals into smaller milestones to make them more achievable.

Create a study schedule that outlines when and what you will study. Allocate time for each content area based on its complexity and importance. Make sure to include dedicated review sessions to reinforce learning and identify areas that require further attention.

Step 3: Use Various Study Resources

Having access to a broad range of materials is essential for effective learning. Utilize textbooks, classroom notes, online resources, and study guides to diversify your knowledge. Invest in a copy of the *"NATIONAL REGISTRY PARAMEDIC PREP"* book, as it provides valuable insights into the exam format and content areas.

Online platforms can offer interactive and engaging learning experiences through quizzes, videos, and discussion forums. Incorporate these resources into your study regimen to solidify concepts and build practical skills.

Step 4: Take Practice Tests & Assess Your Performance

Simulate the exam-taking experience by taking timed practice tests. This will not only help familiarize yourself with the test dynamics but also improve time management skills. Regularly reviewing your test results will give you insight into your progress and pinpoint areas that need improvement.

Study groups can offer additional support by providing feedback on your areas of strength and weakness. Collaborate with peers to exchange information, share experiences, and engage in group discussions.

Step 5: Seek Assistance from Instructors or Mentors

Don't hesitate to ask for help from experienced individuals such as instructors, paramedics, or mentors. Their guidance can provide valuable insight into exam strategies, content nuances, and real-life scenarios.

Step 6: Revisit Topics & Strengthen Weak Areas

Drawing closer to the exam day, identify weak areas and invest more time in reviewing those topics. Strengthening your understanding of problem areas will boost your confidence on the test day.

Step 7: Maintain Physical & Mental Wellness

Preparing for the National Registry Paramedic Exam goes beyond academics—it also requires a holistic approach to wellness. Ensure you are getting enough sleep, regular exercise, proper nutrition, and practicing stress management techniques such as meditation or yoga. A healthy body and mind enhance focus and improve retention of information.

Step 8: Stay Positive & Believe in Yourself

Lastly, maintain a positive attitude throughout the process and have faith in your abilities. Visualize success and embrace challenges as opportunities for growth.

Time Management Techniques

The National Registry Paramedic Exam (NRPE) is an essential milestone for every aspiring paramedic, and it is vital to manage your time efficiently to make the most of your preparation. Below are the effective time management techniques to optimize your study schedule and increase your chances of success on the NRPE.

1. **Set clear goals:** Before you begin studying, outline your objectives for both short-term and long-term achievements. These goals should be specific, measurable, achievable, relevant, and time-bound (SMART). By creating a framework for your progress, you will stay motivated and focused throughout your study journey.

2. **Plan ahead:** Planning is critical when it comes to managing your time effectively. Start by creating a study schedule that outlines how much time you will dedicate per day, week, or month to achieve each goal. Be sure to allocate sufficient time to each subject area covered in the exam and identify areas where you need extra focus.

3. **Prioritize effectively:** While all topics covered in the exam are essential, some require more in-depth knowledge or greater attention than others. Allocate proportionate time to each subject based on your understanding and skills. For instance, if you are weak in cardiology but excel in airway management, you may want to allocate more time to cardiology.

4. **Use effective study techniques:** Finding the right study technique is crucial for optimizing your use of time. Some common productivity-enhancing strategies include:
   - *The Pomodoro Technique:* It involves breaking study sessions into focused 25-minute intervals known as 'pomodoros' with a short break in between. This promotes concentration while reducing mental fatigue.

14

— *Flashcards:* This tool helps reinforce memory through active recall – by reviewing information over an extended period.

— *Practice exams:* Mimic testing conditions and gauge your performance periodically with practice exams.

5. **Avoid procrastination:** Procrastination can be a significant obstacle in preparing for the NRPE. To overcome this, break tasks into manageable smaller pieces. Employ time management techniques, such as setting deadlines or employing the Pomodoro Technique, to maintain consistency and motivation.

6. **Eliminate distractions:** Reduce distractions by creating a comfortable and conducive study environment. Turn off unnecessary notifications on your devices and maintain physical distance from distracting items or people. Inform friends and family of your study schedule and request their cooperation in supporting your efforts.

7. **Rest and recharge:** Giving yourself sufficient rest is crucial to prevent burnout. Ensure you have a regular sleep schedule, engage in physical activity, and set aside time for leisure activities you enjoy. Maintaining a well-balanced routine can boost your overall productivity.

8. **Stay organized:** Keep your study materials in an organized manner – use folders & labels to categorize information by subject or topic area. This system allows you to access resources quickly while avoiding unnecessary waste of time searching for particular documents.

9. **Monitor progress:** Review your progress regularly by conducting self-assessments, timed quizzes, or practice exams. This process helps determine which time management strategies work best for you and identify areas needing improvement. Make adjustments as required to ensure that goals are met within the timeline.

10. **Flexibility:** Your needs may change as you progress through your exam preparation journey; be ready to modify your schedule accordingly. Flexibility in approaching your study plan will ensure that unexpected life events don't throw you off course completely.

Chapter 2

Paramedic Certification Overview

Paramedic certification is an essential milestone for anyone pursuing a career in emergency medical services. Becoming a certified paramedic validates your knowledge, skills, and professional competence to provide advanced life support to patients in emergency situations. One of the most widely recognized certifications is the National Registry Paramedic (NRP) certification, which is administered by the National Registry of Emergency Medical Technicians (NREMT). This chapter provides an overview of the NRP certification process, focusing on understanding the National Registry Paramedic Exam and key concepts and skills assessed.

Understanding the National Registry Paramedic Exam

The path to becoming a certified paramedic is a long and challenging one, but the rewards are worth the effort. One of the most crucial milestones aspiring paramedics must face is passing the National Registry Paramedic (NRP) Exam. Let's help you gain a better understanding of the structure, content, and requirements of this critical assessment, which will be a pivotal step forward in your journey.

The NRP Exam originates from a partnership between numerous organizations, including the National Registry of Emergency Medical Technicians (NREMT) and state licensing agencies, intended to establish consistent standards for EMS certification and licensure. This ensures that certified paramedics possess all necessary skills and knowledge to provide high-quality pre-hospital emergency care, which ultimately translates into lives saved in emergencies.

NRP Exam Structure

The NRP Exam comprises two distinct components: a Computer Adaptive Test (CAT) and a psychomotor skills examination.

1. Computer Adaptive Test (CAT): The CAT consists of between 80 and 150 multiple-choice questions. Candidates have a maximum of 2 hours and 30 minutes to complete this part of the exam. The test adapts to each candidate's responses based on their performance throughout, making for an efficient evaluation of their overall competency. The NREMT utilizes five different content domains within this assessment:

a) Airway Management, Respiration, and Artificial Ventilation
b) Cardiovascular & Medical Emergencies
c) Trauma Emergencies
d) Obstetrics & Pediatrics
e) Operation

Each domain comprises several sub-domains that encompass specific knowledge or capabilities relevant to delivering effective emergency medical care.

2. Psychomotor Skills Examination: While it is essential for aspiring paramedics to possess adequate knowledge and cognitive abilities, their practical skills are equally critical in real-life situations. The psychomotor skills examination evaluates candidates' ability to perform various emergency medical procedures competently. It covers the following essential skill areas:

a) Patient Assessment – Trauma
b) Patient Assessment – Medical
c) Dynamic Cardiology 1 (Cardiac Intervention)
d) Dynamic Cardiology 2 (Management)
e) Pediatric Respiratory Compromise
f) Static Cardiology
g) IV/IO Therapy and Medication Administration

These practical assessments allow testing organizations to confirm the candidate's hands-on competence, attesting to their readiness to perform in actual emergency situations.

Preparing for the NRP Exam

Given that the NRP Exam is designed to test both theoretical knowledge and practical skills, you must dedicate ample time and effort to prepare yourself for success. Here are some strategies to help you tackle the necessary material and boost your chances of passing.

1. **Study Plan:** Organize your studying around the NREMT's content domains and sub-domains, dedicating appropriate time blocks to each topic based on its complexity and relevance.

2. **Diverse Learning Resources:** Utilize a mix of resources such as textbooks, online courses, flashcards, review sheets, video tutorials, and mock exams to maintain engagement throughout your preparation journey.

3. **Hands-on Practice:** Regularly practicing psychomotor skills alongside experienced professionals will help you build muscle memory and confidence crucial for passing the practical examination.

4. **Self-assessment:** Track your progress by taking practice exams simulating the CAT structure and timeline, focusing on areas of weakness that emerge throughout your evaluation.

The Requirements Before & After Passing

Before applying for either component of the NRP exam, aspiring paramedics must have completed an accredited paramedic program within the last two years. Additionally, they need to hold a current Basic Life Support (BLS) credential and Advanced Cardiac Life Support (ACLS) certification.

Once you successfully pass both the cognitive and psychomotor examinations, maintain your NRP certification through regular continuing education and additional recertification examinations conducted every two years.

Key Concepts and Skills Assessed

The National Registry Paramedic (NRP) examination measures the knowledge and skills required to provide prehospital emergency care at an advanced level. This section aims to provide an overview of the key concepts and skills assessed in the NRP examination, ensuring that you are well-prepared for your crucial journey as a paramedic.

The NRP examination evaluates candidates based on five primary domains:

1. Trauma
2. Medical
3. Cardiology
4. Special Considerations
5. Operations

Each of these domains consists of several sub-topics that focus on specific areas of paramedic practice.

1. Trauma: As a paramedic, you will frequently encounter trauma situations requiring assessment and management of various injuries. The NRP examination assesses knowledge and skills in:

- Scene size-up

- Triage
- Primary survey and resuscitation
- Secondary assessment
- Management of specific injuries, such as musculoskeletal, head, spinal, chest and abdominal injuries, as well as burns and soft tissue injuries

2. Medical: Medical emergencies involve complexities beyond those commonly seen in trauma situations. Demonstrating competence in managing these cases is critical to your success on the NRP examination. Topics covered include:

- Assessment and management of respiratory emergencies (COPD, asthma, pneumonia)
- Neurological emergencies (stroke, seizures)
- Abdominal/GI emergencies (appendicitis, pancreatitis)
- Endocrine emergencies (diabetic ketoacidosis)
- Infectious diseases (meningitis, sepsis)
- Environmental hazards (heatstroke, hypothermia)
- Toxicological emergencies (overdose, poisoning)

3. Cardiology: Cardiovascular events represent many life-threatening emergencies that paramedics must be adept at managing. In this domain, the NRP examination focuses on:

- The American Heart Association's BLS and ACLS guidelines
- Interpretation of electrocardiograms (ECGs)
- Assessment and management of various arrhythmias
- Cardiovascular emergencies, such as acute coronary syndromes, heart failure, and cardiogenic shock

4. Special Considerations: Emergencies involving pediatric or geriatric patients, obstetrics, and psychiatric cases require special attention due to differing physiological and psychological needs of the patients. The NRP examination will assess your knowledge and skills in managing these situations:

- Pediatric assessment triangle (PAT)
- Pediatric airway management
- Neonatal resuscitation program (NRP) guidelines
- Geriatric assessment and management, including polypharmacy considerations
- Obstetrical emergencies (delivery complications, postpartum hemorrhage)
- Management of psychosocial issues in emergency care (suicide attempts, agitation)

5. Operations: Effective communication and collaboration are crucial for paramedics to navigate complex prehospital care situations. The NRP examination evaluates your competence in these topics:

- Incident command system
- Communication with medical direction
- Ambulance operations and safety
- Triage systems and mass casualty incident management
- Hazardous materials awareness level knowledge

Beyond the theoretical knowledge of these domains, the NRP examination tests practical skills through scenario-based questions that evaluate clinical decision-making abilities. You must be familiar with specific techniques such as airway management, intravenous therapy administration, medication dosing, defibrillation/cardioversion, and patient assessment.

Additionally, the NRP examination emphasizes critical thinking and ethical considerations involved in paramedic practice. Candidates are expected to prioritize patient safety while adhering to the best practices in delivering care.

Chapter 3

Anatomy, Physiology, Pathophysiology, and Shock

The human body is a complex machine with various systems working together to maintain homeostasis. Paramedics must have a detailed understanding of the anatomy and physiology to recognize when a medical or traumatic injury occurs and provide effective emergency care. This chapter explores the human body systems, pathophysiology, shock, and essential concepts for paramedics.

The Human Body Systems

The human body is an intricate and complex network of systems that work together to maintain homeostasis and promote overall health. In this chapter, we will explore the different body systems and their importance in maintaining a healthy functioning body. As a paramedic, it is essential to understand these systems to effectively respond to medical emergencies and provide essential care.

1. **The Integumentary System:** The integumentary system consists of the skin, hair, nails, and other accessory structures that offer protection, regulation, and sensation. The skin is the largest organ of the body, protecting the internal organs from injury or infection. It also helps regulate body temperature through sweating and shivering. Additionally, the integumentary system serves as a physical barrier to harmful radiation and chemicals, while also providing sensory information about the external environment.

2. **The Musculoskeletal System:** The musculoskeletal system includes bones, joints, muscles, tendons, ligaments, cartilage, and other connective tissue. This system provides support for the body and offers protection for vital organs. The muscles are responsible

for movement within each joint by contracting or expanding as necessary. The musculoskeletal system also plays a key role in maintaining posture and balance.

3. **The Nervous System:** Composed of the brain, spinal cord, nerves, ganglia, sensory organs like eyes and ears, the nervous system serves as the body's control center. It provides rapid communication and coordination among all other systems via electrical impulses transmitted through neurons. The nervous system can be divided into two main parts: the central nervous system (CNS), comprising the brain and spinal cord; and the peripheral nervous system (PNS), connecting CNS to all other body parts.

4. **The Cardiovascular System:** The cardiovascular system comprises the heart (a muscular pump), blood vessels (arteries, veins, and capillaries), and blood. It functions to transport oxygen, nutrients, hormones, waste products, and other important substances throughout the body. Maintaining healthy blood pressure and preventing cardiovascular disease are essential tasks for paramedics when responding to medical emergencies.

5. **The Respiratory System:** Encompassing the nose, mouth, pharynx, larynx, trachea, bronchi, and lungs, the respiratory system is responsible for delivering oxygen to the body and eliminating carbon dioxide and other waste gases. Respiration is a vital process that influences many aspects of a patient's health and many medical emergencies are related to this system.

6. **The Digestive System:** The digestive system is responsible for breaking down food into simple nutrients that can be absorbed into the bloodstream. This system includes organs such as the mouth, esophagus, stomach, small intestine, large intestine, rectum, pancreas, liver, and gallbladder. It also plays an essential role in maintaining proper fluid balance and electrolyte levels.

7. **The Urinary System:** The urinary system filters waste products from the bloodstream and eliminates them via urine production. It includes organs like kidneys (two bean-shaped organs), ureters (small tubes connecting kidneys to bladder), urinary bladder (reservoir for urine storage), and urethra (tube leading outside body). Proper hydration is crucial for maintaining a healthy urinary system since dehydration can hinder its function.

8. **The Endocrine System:** This system consists of several glands that produce hormones responsible for regulating various physiological processes such as growth, metabolism, reproductive health, stress response, and more. Some major endocrine glands include the hypothalamus (pituitary gland's link to the brain), pituitary (adrenal glands' stimulator), thyroid (regulates metabolism), parathyroid (calcium balance maintenance), adrenal (essential in fight or flight response) glands; genitals.

9. **The Reproductive System:** Involving the organs and tissues involved in producing offspring, the reproductive system also contains vital hormones, which impact not just reproduction but overall health and wellness. Testes in males and ovaries in females are responsible for producing sperm and eggs, respectively. Proper awareness of male and female reproductive health issues can help ensure timely intervention during medical emergencies.

10. **The Lymphatic System:** Comprising lymph nodes, vessels, tonsils, spleen, and thymus gland, the lymphatic system works concurrently with the cardiovascular system to filter harmful substances from tissues, retain interstitial fluid balance and preserve immunity.

Pathophysiology

Pathophysiology is the study of disordered physiological processes that cause, result from, or are otherwise associated with diseases or injuries. As a paramedic, understanding the underlying principles of pathophysiology is crucial for effective treatment and management of patients with various medical conditions.

To begin, it is important to distinguish between disease etiology and pathogenesis. Etiology refers to the factors that contribute to the development of a disease, while pathogenesis describes the process by which a disease progresses. These two components play crucial roles in determining a patient's symptoms and treatment options.

One of the foundational concepts in pathophysiology is inflammation. Inflammation is the body's natural response to injury or infection and serves to facilitate tissue repair and prevent further damage. It typically involves redness, heat, swelling, pain, and sometimes loss of function in the affected area. Although inflammation is initially helpful in promoting healing, chronic inflammation can lead to tissue damage, impaired function, and long-term complications.

The immune system plays a vital role in defending the body against foreign substances and organisms like bacteria, viruses, or other pathogens. Under normal conditions, immune cells recognize and destroy potentially harmful substances before they can cause damage. However, when the immune system becomes unbalanced—either too weak or too strong—it can result in increased susceptibility to infections or autoimmune diseases like lupus or rheumatoid arthritis.

Shock is an essential concept for paramedics in understanding how the body responds to severe injury or illness. Shock occurs when there is insufficient blood flow (perfusion) to meet the body's oxygen and nutrient demands. This can result from several factors such as low blood volume (hypovolemic shock), poor heart function (cardiogenic shock), excessive blood vessel dilation (distributive shock), or a combination of these factors (multiple etiology shock). Rapid identification and correct treatment of shock are vital for improving patient outcomes.

In addition to these overarching concepts, paramedics should be familiar with a variety of disease processes that can affect individual organs or organ systems. For example:

- Cardiac pathophysiology covers conditions such as ischemic heart disease, myocardial infarction (heart attack), congestive heart failure, and arrhythmias. Understanding cardiac physiology allows paramedics to recognize the signs and symptoms of these conditions and initiate appropriate treatment in the prehospital setting.

- Respiratory pathophysiology encompasses diseases that impact the lungs and airways, including chronic obstructive pulmonary disease (COPD), bronchitis, pneumonia, asthma, and pulmonary embolism. Paramedics must identify symptoms suggestive of respiratory distress or failure and provide necessary interventions to improve breathing.

- Neuropathophysiology involves the study of neurological disorders like stroke (cerebrovascular accident), traumatic brain injury, seizures, and spinal cord injuries. Prompt recognition of neurological deficits by paramedics is crucial for early intervention and reducing the risk of long-term complications in patients.

- Endocrine pathophysiology examines the influence of hormones and hormonal imbalances on health. Conditions like diabetes mellitus, thyroid disorders, and adrenal insufficiency are examples of endocrine diseases that can profoundly affect a patient's physiological state. Emergency medical professionals must be equipped to manage these medical emergencies appropriately.

- Gastrointestinal pathophysiology deals with conditions affecting the digestive system, such as gastroesophageal reflux disease (GERD), peptic ulcers, inflammatory bowel disease (IBD), and obstruction. As a paramedic, you must be able to recognize signs of GI distress and provide proper relief or stabilization for your patient until definitive care can be given.

The study of pathophysiology is complex and ongoing as new research continually advances our understanding of disease processes. As a paramedic, staying up-to-date with the latest evidence-based practices is key to providing effective care for your patients. Ultimately, a strong foundation in pathophysiology empowers you to make informed decisions during high-pressure situations and contribute positively to the overall health and well-being of the communities you serve.

Shock

Shock is a critical and life-threatening condition encountered by paramedics during emergency situations. It is a result of inadequate perfusion, causing inadequate oxygen delivery to the body's tissues and cells. Let's discuss the different types of shock, their pathophysiology, signs and symptoms, and management strategies employed by paramedics to reverse the state of shock.

1. **Hypovolemic Shock:** Hypovolemic shock is the most common form of shock that occurs due to low blood volume resulting from blood loss, dehydration, or a combination of both factors. Blood loss can be caused by trauma, surgery, internal hemorrhage, or burns.

2. **Cardiogenic Shock:** Cardiogenic shock occurs when the heart fails to pump blood effectively due to myocardial damage or dysfunction. The causes include myocardial infarction (heart attack), cardiac arrhythmias, myocarditis (inflammation of the heart muscle), cardiomyopathy (a weakened heart muscle), or valvular disease.

3. **Distributive Shock:** Distributive shock results from an imbalance in vascular tone leading to increased capillary permeability and vasodilation. This type of shock can be further categorized into three subtypes: septic shock, neurogenic shock, and anaphylactic

shock.

a) *Septic Shock* - Septic shock is caused by an overwhelming bacterial infection that leads to a systemic inflammatory response.

b) *Neurogenic Shock* - Neurogenic shock results from spinal cord injury or damage affecting autonomic nervous system regulation.

c) *Anaphylactic Shock* - Anaphylactic shock is an extreme allergic reaction causing widespread release of histamine leading to vasodilation and capillary leakage.

4. **Obstructive Shock:** Obstructive shock occurs when a physical obstruction impedes blood flow through the circulatory system. The most common causes include tension pneumothorax, cardiac tamponade, and pulmonary embolism.

Signs and Symptoms

In general, signs and symptoms of shock include:

— Altered level of consciousness or confusion

— Tachycardia (rapid heart rate) or bradycardia (slow heart rate) in the case of neurogenic shock

— Hypotension (low blood pressure)

— Pale, cool, and clammy skin

— Rapid, shallow breathing or respiratory distress

— Weak and thready pulse

— Oliguria (reduced urine output)

— Delayed capillary refill time with cyanosis

Paramedic Management

The primary goals of paramedic interventions in shock are to restore tissue perfusion, optimize oxygen delivery, and prevent further damage. Some general strategies are:

1. **Airway management:** Maintaining a patent airway and ensuring proper ventilation is vital. Administer high-flow oxygen via non-rebreather masks, provide assisted ventilations with a bag-valve mask if necessary, or employ advanced airway techniques.

2. **Fluid resuscitation:** For hypovolemic shock or distributive shock (except neurogenic), rapid fluid resuscitation is recommended using isotonic crystalloid solutions like normal saline or lactated Ringer's solution at 20ml/kg. In neurogenic shock, smaller volumes may be used together with vasoconstrictors to balance the risk of exacerbating hypotension.

3. **Vasoactive medications:** Vasoactive medications like epinephrine, norepinephrine, dopamine, or vasopressin may be administered through intravenous (IV) or intraosseous (IO) access to support blood pressure and cardiac output.

4. **Hemostasis:** Control any external hemorrhage using direct pressure, tourniquets, hemostatic gauze or wound packing.

5. **Rapid transport:** If shock is suspected, rapid and safe transport to a definitive care facility is essential. During transport, closely monitor the patient's vital signs, including heart rate, blood pressure, respiratory rate, and level of consciousness.

Essential Concepts for Paramedics

Aspiring paramedics must understand a variety of essential concepts to be successful in their career. These key principles play a crucial role in the effective and efficient delivery of prehospital care by paramedics during emergency situations. Let's focus on these vital concepts and how they are applied in the daily practice of a paramedic.

1. **Assessment and Triage:** One of the most crucial aspects of being a paramedic is knowing how to perform an accurate assessment. This task involves quickly gauging the condition of a patient by evaluating their vital signs and gathering relevant medical history. An organized approach ensures that important information is not overlooked, which is crucial in providing appropriate care.
Triage, on the other hand, involves deciding which patients require immediate attention and prioritizing them based on severity. This step is particularly important during mass casualty incidents when multiple patients need treatment simultaneously.

2. **Airway Management:** Airway management is a fundamental skill for any paramedic. Maintaining an open airway is necessary for ensuring adequate oxygenation and ventilation of patients. Various techniques exist for managing airway obstructions, ranging from simple maneuvers (e.g., head tilt-chin lift) to advanced interventions (e.g., endotracheal intubation). Familiarity with these techniques allows paramedics to act decisively and rapidly in emergencies.

3. **Circulation Support:** Effective circulation support involves understanding the cardiovascular system and its role in providing oxygen and nutrients to vital organs. Paramedics must recognize signs of circulatory failure, such as hypotension or unresponsiveness, and administer appropriate treatment accordingly (e.g., CPR, defibrillation).

4. **Trauma Management:** Paramedics encounter traumatic injuries frequently, making trauma management an indispensable skill. Key components include primary and secondary surveys, immobilization techniques for fractures, control of bleeding through direct pressure or tourniquet application, and recognition of internal injuries that may necessitate rapid transport to a trauma center.

5. **Pharmacology:** Paramedics must possess an in-depth knowledge of the drugs they administer and their potential effects on patients. This understanding includes proper dosages, contraindications, side effects, and drug interactions. Additionally, paramedics should be prepared to recognize and manage any adverse reactions that may arise during drug administration.

6. **Medical Emergencies:** Many medical emergencies (e.g., stroke, myocardial infarction) require immediate recognition and intervention by paramedics. They must be able to differentiate between various conditions, utilizing assessment skills and knowledge of relevant pharmacology to initiate appropriate treatment protocols. Rapid decision-making may greatly improve patient outcomes, making this skill especially valuable in emergency medical services.

7. **Effective Communication:** Paramedics work closely with other healthcare professionals (e.g., nurses, physicians) during patient care and handovers; therefore, clear and concise communication is essential. This skill ensures that accurate information is exchanged and transmitted to the receiving facility while minimizing potential errors or misunderstandings.

8. **Emotional Resilience:** Working as a paramedic can be both mentally and physically demanding. Responding to high-stress situations may cause psychological strain, making emotional resilience a crucial trait for a successful paramedic career. Learning how to cope with stressors and seeking support when needed helps maintain mental health and fosters appropriate patient care.

9. **Professionalism:** Paramedics represent their profession's values through professionalism in their day-to-day interactions with patients, colleagues, family members, and bystanders. Ethical decision-making plays a significant role in this aspect, underlining the importance of maintaining patient confidentiality and adhering to legal parameters while providing care.

10. **Continuing Education:** Advancements in medical knowledge occur perpetually; thus, a commitment to lifelong learning is vital for any paramedic aiming to maintain competence in their ever-evolving profession. Participating in continuing education courses, staying current with the latest research, and engaging in clinical practice guideline updates ensure that paramedics remain effective providers in their field.

Chapter 4

Cardiology and Resuscitation

The cardiovascular system is composed of the heart, blood vessels, and blood. The heart is a muscular organ that pumps blood throughout the body via a network of blood vessels consisting of arteries, capillaries, and veins. The main function of this system is to transport oxygen, nutrients, hormones, and waste products to and from different cells and tissues within the body.

The heart itself is divided into four chambers: two atria (upper chambers) and two ventricles (lower chambers). Blood enters the right atrium from systemic circulation through the superior and inferior vena cavae. It then passes through the tricuspid valve into the right ventricle before being pumped through the pulmonary valve into pulmonary circulation via pulmonary arteries. Oxygenation occurs in capillaries surrounding alveoli within the lungs. Oxygen-rich blood returns to the left atrium via pulmonary veins then flows through the bicuspid or mitral valve into the left ventricle. Finally, it is propelled through the aortic valve into systemic circulation via the aorta.

Understanding these anatomical structures will assist in identifying cardiovascular pathologies and selecting appropriate treatment modalities in paramedic practice.

Cardiac Rhythm Interpretation

One crucial aspect of cardiology for paramedics is cardiac rhythm interpretation. Paramedics should be proficient in recognizing normal sinus rhythm as well as various forms of arrhythmias such as atrial fibrillation, atrial flutter, ventricular tachycardia, ventricular fibrillation, and asystole. They should also be familiar with atrioventricular (AV) blocks and pace-maker rhythms.

Establishing an accurate rhythm diagnosis is vital to direct appropriate cardiac pharmacological interventions and electrical therapies including cardioversion and defibrillation.

Acute Coronary Syndrome

Acute coronary syndrome (ACS) is a term used to describe situations where blood supply to the heart muscle is blocked, leading to chest pain (angina), myocardial infarction (heart attack), or other complications. Paramedics should be skilled in the rapid assessment of patients presenting with possible ACS symptoms, including obtaining a thorough history and physical examination along with acquiring and interpreting electrocardiograms (ECGs).

Prompt identification and early intervention can significantly reduce morbidity and mortality rates associated with ACS. Treatment options include administering oxygen therapy, nitroglycerin, aspirin, beta-blockers, anticoagulants, analgesics as well as providing emotional support to the patient.

Cardiopulmonary Resuscitation (CPR)

Cardiopulmonary resuscitation (CPR) is a vital life-saving technique that all paramedics should master. CPR involves the combination of chest compressions and rescue breaths to maintain circulation and oxygenation in cardiac arrest patients. High-quality CPR is crucial for improving survival rates and overall neurological outcomes in those experiencing cardiac arrest.

Paramedics should stay up-to-date on the latest guidelines issued by the American Heart Association to ensure they are utilizing the most effective CPR techniques.

Advanced Cardiac Life Support (ACLS)

Advanced Cardiac Life Support (ACLS) encompasses various medical interventions targeting the management of cardiac arrest beyond basic life support measures. ACLS includes airway management, intravenous access establishment, administration of emergency medications, and electrical therapies like defibrillation and pacing.

Paramedics should become proficient in identifying indications for specific ACLS interventions and exercising effective communication in organizing the resuscitation team.

Chapter 5

Medical Emergencies

M edical emergencies are situations that require immediate medical attention in order to prevent severe harm or death. These emergencies can occur unexpectedly and often require rapid assessment, management, and treatment by skilled responders. Paramedics are often at the forefront of handling these situations, and they need to be prepared for a wide range of scenarios that can arise. In this chapter, we will take a closer look at some of the most common medical emergencies that paramedics encounter, in order to provide a comprehensive resource for those who serve as first responders on the frontlines of emergency medical care.

Cardiac and Respiratory Emergencies

An understanding of the basic anatomy and physiology of the heart is necessary to effectively manage cardiac emergencies. The heart is responsible for pumping oxygenated blood throughout the body, providing essential nutrients to tissues. It comprises four chambers - two atria (upper chambers) which receive blood, and two ventricles (lower chambers) that pump blood.

Blood circulation consists of two loops; pulmonary circulation that involves blood flow between the heart and lungs for oxygenation, and systemic circulation carrying oxygenated blood to tissues throughout the body. Regulation of heart function occurs through intricate electrical conduction systems involving sinoatrial (SA) node, atrioventricular (AV) node, bundle of His, bundle branches, and Purkinje fibers.

Common Cardiac Emergencies

Cardiac emergencies encompass a wide range of conditions arising from the heart's malfunction or structural anomalies. These can include acute coronary syndromes (ACS), arrhythmias, and palpitations.

1. Acute Coronary Syndromes (ACS): ACS is a spectrum of conditions under which blood supply to the heart muscle is reduced or blocked. ACS includes unstable angina, non-ST elevation myocardial infarction (NSTEMI), and ST-elevation myocardial infarction (STEMI).

Key signs and symptoms of ACS include:

- Chest pain or discomfort
- Pain radiating to the arms, neck, jaw, shoulders, or back
- Shortness of breath
- Nausea
- Sweating
- Weakness

Paramedics should administer oxygen if patients have hypoxia or signs of heart failure. Administer aspirin to inhibit platelet aggregation unless contraindicated. Nitroglycerin can be used if prescribed to relieve chest pain. It is crucial to transport patients experiencing ACS promptly to a medical facility.

2. Arrhythmias: Arrhythmias are abnormalities in the heart rhythm that can cause it to pump less effectively. Examples include atrial fibrillation (AF), atrioventricular blocks, and ventricular fibrillation (VF).

Symptoms associated with arrhythmias include:

- Palpitations
- Dizziness or lightheadedness
- Fatigue
- Chest pain

To manage arrhythmias, follow ACLS guidelines appropriate for specific arrhythmias. Maintain airway, breathing, and circulation (ABC) and administer appropriate medications as prescribed.

Common Respiratory Emergencies

Respiratory emergencies occur due to the failure of the respiratory system to maintain adequate oxygenation and ventilation. Some common conditions include chronic obstructive pulmonary disease (COPD), asthma, pneumonia, and pulmonary embolism.

1. Chronic Obstructive Pulmonary Disease (COPD): COPD refers to a group of lung diseases characterized by obstructed airflow, primarily caused by smoking. Symptoms include shortness of breath, coughing, wheezing, and excess mucus production.

To manage COPD exacerbations, administer supplemental oxygen if needed, noninvasive positive pressure ventilation (NIPPV), and bronchodilator medications such as ipratropium bromide/albuterol (Duoneb).

2. Asthma: Asthma is a chronic inflammatory condition characterized by constricted airway passages and excessive mucus production. Triggers include allergens, physical activities, and stress.

During an asthma attack, paramedics should provide supplemental oxygen if needed, inhaled bronchodilators like albuterol or levalbuterol, and intramuscular epinephrine for severe exacerbations.

3. Pneumonia: Pneumonia is an infection that causes inflammation in the lungs' air sacs. Symptoms include fever, cough with mucus production, chest pain during breaths or coughs, and shortness of breath.

Paramedics should administer supplemental oxygen if required and transport the patient to the hospital for further assessment and treatment.

4. Pulmonary Embolism: Pulmonary embolism is a blood clot that travels through the bloodstream into the lungs' pulmonary arteries. This can cause life-threatening respiratory distress if not treated promptly.

Symptoms of pulmonary embolism may include:

-   Sudden, unexplained shortness of breath
-   Chest pain, especially when breathing deeply or coughing
-   Palpitations

Paramedic management includes supplemental oxygen, intravenous (IV) line establishment, and alerting the receiving facility of possible pulmonary embolism.

Neurological and Gastrointestinal Emergencies

Neurological and gastrointestinal emergencies are common occurrences that require prompt recognition and intervention by paramedics. As a paramedic, understanding the pathophysiology of these emergencies is crucial to identifying and managing patients presenting with neurological or gastrointestinal conditions in the field.

This section will provide a comprehensive overview of key concepts, assessments, and treatments for these types of emergencies, helping you to successfully navigate and prepare for the challenges you may face in the National Registry Paramedic Exam.

Common Neurological Emergencies

Neurological emergencies can stem from various factors, including head trauma, cerebrovascular accidents (CVAs), seizures, infections, and other medical conditions. Below are the most common neurological emergencies that paramedics may encounter.

1. Head Trauma: Head trauma is a common cause of neurological dysfunction and may result from falls, motor vehicle accidents, assaults, or sports-related injuries. Paramedics should assess airway, breathing and circulation (ABCs), obtain Glasgow Coma Scale (GCS) scores to evaluate the severity of head injury and monitor vital signs carefully.

Pain control should be provided while minimizing agitation or unnecessary stimulation. Maintain adequate oxygenation and ventilation with supplemental oxygen or assist controlled ventilation as needed. In cases of penetrating head injuries or suspected skull fractures, apply occlusive dressings while maintaining cervical spine precautions.

2. CVAs (strokes): Cerebrovascular accidents or strokes occur when blood flow to the brain is disrupted due to blockage or rupturing of blood vessels. Common signs include sudden onset severe headache, facial droop, slurred speech, arm drift or weakness on one side of the body.

Immediate transport to appropriate stroke care facilities is essential for administration of clot-busting medications before irreversible brain damage occurs. In any suspected stroke patient always maintain airway and support adequate oxygenation as necessary.

3. Seizures: Seizure disorders have multiple causes such as epilepsy, alcohol or drug withdrawal, brain tumors, or electrolyte imbalances. Paramedics should observe the duration and description of seizure activity to help guide treatment.

The primary goal is to protect the patient and bystanders and maintain airway security. When managing discontinuous seizures, consider administering benzodiazepines (e.g., midazolam, lorazepam) to reduce seizure activity. In prolonged seizures, proper medical management may be necessary.

Common Gastrointestinal Emergencies

Gastrointestinal emergencies involve disturbances in the GI tract functions, which include ingestion, digestion, absorption, and elimination of solid waste. Some common gastrointestinal emergencies are discussed below.

1. Abdominal Pain: Abdominal pain can arise from many conditions like gastrointestinal infection, bowel obstruction, pancreatitis, gastritis, post-operative complications or appendicitis. Paramedics should obtain a thorough history and look for any red flag symptoms to direct further evaluation.

Ensure the patient is comfortable with elevating their legs if necessary. In cases of severe pain, consider providing analgesia as per local protocols. Monitor vital signs closely and transport the patient to an appropriate medical facility.

2. Gastrointestinal Bleeding: GI bleeding may occur due to inflammation in the upper (esophagus, stomach, or upper intestine) or lower (colon) GI tract in conditions like ulcers or diverticular disease. Patients may present with hematemesis or melena (dark-colored feces).

Management focuses on maintaining a patent airway, administering oxygen as necessary, careful monitoring of vital signs and adequate intravenous fluid resuscitation as patients can quickly become hemodynamically unstable.

3. Bowel Obstruction: Bowel obstructions might result from adhesions inside the abdominal cavity due to previous surgery or inflammation causing twisting or kinking of the bowels. Symptoms include severe abdominal pain, distension, nausea/vomiting, and obstipation (severe constipation).

Provide pain control as per local guidelines and administer antiemetics for nausea when indicated. Evaluate patient's hydration status carefully, as dehydration may develop rapidly due to vomiting and fluid sequestration within the obstructed bowels.

Obstetrics and Gynecology Emergencies

Obstetrics and gynecological emergencies require prompt recognition and management, as both the mother and the fetus's lives could be at risk. Paramedics must be prepared to handle these situations efficiently and effectively to ensure optimal outcomes for both the mother and the fetus.

1. **Labor and Delivery Complications:** Labor and delivery is a complex process with several potential complications that paramedics need to be familiar with. These complications can include prolonged or arrested labor, breech presentation, cord prolapse, placental abruption, and uterine rupture.

   a) *Prolonged or Arrested Labor:* Labor may take longer than expected or might not progress at all. If the cervix does not dilate adequately or contractions are ineffective in moving the baby through the birth canal, this may lead to prolonged or arrested labor. Paramedics should seek medical direction for managing pain and preparing for transport in these situations.

   b) *Breech Presentation:* Breech presentation occurs when the fetus's buttocks or feet enter the birth canal first instead of its head. Paramedics should not attempt to deliver a breech baby in the field unless absolutely unavoidable as it can lead to serious complications for both the mother and fetus.

   c) *Cord Prolapse:* Umbilical cord prolapse is when the umbilical cord descends ahead of the baby through the birth canal during labor. Paramedics must recognize this emergency quickly, as it can cause oxygen deprivation to the fetus if not addressed immediately.

   d) *Placental Abruption:* In some cases, the placenta starts to prematurely detach from the uterus' wall before delivery occurs, causing abdominal pain and heavy vaginal bleeding. Paramedics should consider the possibility of placental abruption in patients with these symptoms, stabilize the patient as much as possible, and expedite transportation to a hospital.

   e) *Uterine Rupture:* Uterine rupture is a rare but life-threatening event where the uterus tears open during labor. Paramedics need to consider this possibility when there is no improvement or increasing pain during contractions, even without bleeding, and transport the patient promptly to the closest facility capable of managing this emergency.

2. **Obstetric Hemorrhage:** Heavy vaginal bleeding during pregnancy can result from various causes. It is essential to differentiate between life-threatening conditions that require immediate intervention, such as uterine rupture or placental abruption, and non-life-threatening situations, such as spotting or bloody show during usual labor. Paramedics should maintain strict infection control practices when managing these patients and prepare for fluid resuscitation and rapid transport as needed.

3. **Ectopic Pregnancy:** An ectopic pregnancy occurs when an embryo implants outside the uterus, typically within a fallopian tube. Women may experience lower abdominal pain, vaginal bleeding, or even shock if there is significant internal bleeding due to a ruptured ectopic pregnancy. The patient should be managed for shock, provided with high-flow oxygen and fluid resuscitation if necessary, and transported immediately for surgical intervention.

4. **Pelvic Inflammatory Disease (PID):** Pelvic inflammatory disease (PID) is an infection of the female reproductive organs that may result in long-term complications such as chronic pain or infertility if left untreated. PID presents with lower abdominal pain, fever, abnormal vaginal discharge, and sometimes nausea and vomiting. Paramedics must manage the patient's pain levels carefully and transport them to a medical facility for further diagnostic testing and antibiotic treatment.

5. **Toxic Shock Syndrome (TSS):** Toxic shock syndrome (TSS) is a rare but severe complication caused by toxin-producing strains of Staphylococcus aureus or Streptococcus pyogenes and usually affects menstruating women using tampons. Symptoms include sudden high fever, hypotension, rash resembling sunburn, vomiting, diarrhea, and mental status changes. It is essential to recognize this syndrome early and provide supportive care, including aggressive fluid resuscitation, oxygen, and transporting the patient to an appropriate medical facility.

Chapter 6

Gynecology, Obstetrics, and Newborn Resuscitation

Gynecology and Obstetrics are two essential branches of medical science that focus on the health and reproductive systems of women throughout their lifetime. As a paramedic, it is vital to understand the essential principles of these fields when attending to prenatal and obstetric emergencies. In this chapter, we will discuss gynecology and obstetrics in detail, followed by essential information on newborn resuscitation for effective National Registry Paramedic preparation.

Gynecology

Gynecology is a branch that focuses on the health of the female reproductive system. As paramedics, it is essential to understand the basic concepts of gynecology to provide appropriate prehospital care for female patients.

The female reproductive system consists of internal and external structures, each having vital functions for reproduction. The primary internal organs include the ovaries, fallopian tubes, uterus, cervix, and vagina. External structures involve the labia majora and minora, clitoris, and Bartholin's glands. Familiarity with these structures and their purpose is crucial when assessing and managing gynecological emergencies.

Several common gynecological conditions may present with discomfort or pain that requires paramedic intervention. Some examples include:

1. **Dysmenorrhea:** This term refers to menstrual cramps or pain occurring during

menstruation due to prostaglandin release, causing uterine contractions.

2. **Menorrhagia:** Heavy or prolonged menstrual bleeding can lead to anemia and hypovolemia if not appropriately managed.

3. **Polycystic Ovary Syndrome (PCOS):** A hormonal imbalance causes multiple cysts on the ovaries, irregular periods, and other symptoms such as excess hair growth or weight gain.

4. **Endometriosis:** Endometrial tissue grows outside the uterus causing severe pain and infertility in some cases.

5. **Uterine Fibroids:** These non-cancerous tumors grow in or around the uterus causing heavy bleeding or pelvic pressure and pain.

Paramedics should be familiar with various gynecological emergencies like ectopic pregnancies, spontaneous abortions (miscarriages), and pelvic inflammatory disease (PID). Early recognition of these conditions can significantly impact the patient's outcome and should be reported immediately to the receiving facility for further management.

Ectopic pregnancies occur when a fertilized egg implants outside the uterus, most commonly in the fallopian tube. Patients may present with abdominal pain, vaginal bleeding, and dizziness or syncope due to intra-abdominal bleeding. Emergency treatment includes IV fluids, supplemental oxygen, monitoring vital signs, and rapid transport for surgical intervention.

Spontaneous abortions, or miscarriages, are the loss of pregnancy before the 20th week. Experiences include pain and bleeding depending on gestational age when loss occurs. Key prehospital care considerations involve pain management, emotional support, and assessing for signs of sepsis or hemorrhage.

Pelvic inflammatory disease (PID) is an infection of female reproductive organs caused by bacteria such as Chlamydia or Gonorrhea. Symptoms include lower abdominal pain, fever, and abnormal vaginal discharge. Management involves administering analgesics for pain relief, monitoring vital signs, and transport to a receiving facility for further care.

Additional pertinent information that should be elicited includes pertinent elements such as the patient's last menstrual period (LMP), whether currently using contraception (type and duration), previous gynecological or obstetrical history as it pertains to their current presentation.

Obstetrics

Obstetrics is a critical branch of medicine that deals with pregnancy, childbirth, and postpartum care. As a paramedic, you play an essential role in providing medical care to expectant mothers, newborns, and their families during these crucial life events.

One of the most important principles in obstetrics is antenatal care, which involves regular monitoring of a pregnant woman's health throughout her pregnancy. This includes assessing maternal vital signs and fetal well-being, testing for pre-existing medical conditions or other potential issues, identifying signs of complications such as gestational diabetes or preeclampsia, and ensuring the expectant mother attends regular prenatal check-ups.

Paramedics should thoroughly understand the three stages of labor as these stages determine appropriate interventions and management:

1. **First stage:** The cervix dilates from 0 cm to 10 cm due to uterine contractions. This stage is further divided into the latent phase (0-3 cm) and active phase (4-10 cm). Labor typically lasts from 6 to 12 hours for first-time mothers and progresses more quickly for those who have previously given birth.

2. **Second stage:** This stage begins when the cervix is fully dilated at 10 cm and ends with the delivery of the baby. It usually lasts from 20 minutes to two hours and involves pushing efforts by the mother.

3. **Third stage:** After birth, this stage involves the delivery of the placenta (afterbirth) within 5-30 minutes.

During labor and delivery, emergencies can arise that require rapid assessment and intervention on behalf of paramedics:

1. **Prolapsed cord:** If the umbilical cord descends ahead of or alongside the baby's head, it can be compressed between the baby's head and the cervix or vagina, cutting off blood flow and oxygen to the baby. Paramedics must recognize this emergency and assist in repositioning the mother, administering oxygen, and, if possible, manually elevating the baby's head off the cord.

2. **Breech presentation:** The baby is delivered buttocks-first instead of head-first. Paramedics should avoid attempting vaginal delivery in this situation and opt for rapid transportation to a medical facility.

3. **Shoulder dystocia:** The baby's head is delivered, but one or both shoulders become stuck behind the mother's pelvic bones. Applying suprapubic pressure or performing the McRoberts maneuver may help facilitate delivery.

In emergency childbirth situations, paramedics should be prepared to manage common neonatal complications:

1. **Neonatal resuscitation:** Approximately 10% of newborns require some resuscitative efforts immediately after birth. This often involves the use of suctioning, bag-mask ventilation, chest compressions, and appropriate medication administration per current guidelines.

2. **Meconium aspiration syndrome:** Meconium-stained amniotic fluid can lead to airway obstruction or infection, requiring early suctioning and ongoing respiratory support.

3. **Hypothermia:** Maintain normal body temperature by promoting skin-to-skin contact between mother and baby or using external heat sources.

Postpartum hemorrhage (PPH) is another potential complication that requires prompt recognition and management. PPH occurs when a woman loses more than 500 ml of blood after delivery. Interventions include uterine massage to stimulate contractions, administering uterotonic medications, IV fluid resuscitation, and rapid transportation to a hospital setting for definitive care.

Newborn Resuscitation

The process of newborn resuscitation plays a critical role in neonatal care and is essential knowledge for paramedics, especially those working in the pre-hospital setting. Newborn resuscitation is a life-saving intervention performed when a newborn exhibits signs of respiratory distress or is not breathing at birth. The importance of prompt and effective resuscitation cannot be overstated, as delayed or inadequate efforts can result in irreversible damage to the newborn's brain, heart, and other organs.

A key aspect of any resuscitation effort is identifying the need for intervention. Paramedics must assess the newborn for signs of respiratory distress or absence of spontaneous breathing. The Apgar scoring system is often used as an initial evaluation tool to determine if further interventions are needed. The Apgar score assesses five critical parameters: appearance, pulse, grimace, activity, and respiration. A score below 7 indicates that the newborn requires assistance.

The equipment used during newborn resuscitation should include an appropriately sized self-inflating bag with a reservoir and positive-force-valve (PFV), an oxygen source with a blender capable of providing precise FiO2 levels ranging from 21% to 100%, a functioning suction device with flexible tubing and sterile suction catheters, pulse oximeter for continuous monitoring of oxygen saturation (SpO2), endotracheal tubes for advanced airway management if required, and a radiant warmer or other appropriate means to maintain the newborn's body temperature.

Once the need for resuscitation is identified, the following steps should be taken:

1. Place the newborn on a flat surface under a radiant warmer or on an open bed with appropriate heat preservation.
2. Suction the airway using a bulb syringe or suction catheter to remove any secretions.
3. Provide 30 seconds of positive pressure ventilation (PPV), ensuring proper mask seal and optimal respiratory rate.
4. Assess the newborn's heart rate and initiate chest compressions if it is below 60 beats per minute.
5. Maintain continuous SpO2 monitoring, aiming for an oxygen saturation target of 90% to 95%.
6. If required, consider establishing an advanced airway through intubation or placement of a laryngeal mask airway (LMA).
7. Administer medications such as epinephrine if needed, as directed by your local protocols and guidelines.

It is crucial that paramedics follow updated guidelines provided by the American Heart

42

Association (AHA), International Liaison Committee on Resuscitation (ILCOR), or other governing bodies to deliver evidence-based care during newborn resuscitation.

Chapter 7

Trauma and Injury Management

Trauma and injury management is a vital aspect of prehospital emergency care. The swift and accurate identification, assessment, and treatment of traumatic injuries are critical to improving patient outcomes and preventing further complications. As a paramedic, you will encounter various types of trauma in the field, ranging from minor injuries to life-threatening emergencies. Understanding the principles of trauma management and being skilled in assessing and treating fractures, burns, soft tissue injuries, and other medical emergencies is crucial for saving lives. In this chapter, we provide an overview of trauma assessment and triage while addressing common types of injuries such as fractures, burns, and soft tissue injuries.

Trauma Assessment and Triage

In this section, we will discuss the process of trauma assessment and triage, important components of a paramedic's role in providing emergency care. Learning how to accurately assess and triage trauma patients is crucial for any aspiring National Registry Paramedic. We will cover the steps involved in trauma assessment, important indicators for injury severity, and the guidelines for triaging patients in emergencies.

1. **Primary Assessment:** Upon arriving at the scene, a primary assessment is conducted to quickly identify life-threatening injuries or conditions. This comprises scene safety, body substance isolation (BSI), determining the mechanism of injury (MOI) or nature of illness (NOI), evaluating mental status using acute stroke scale (AVPU), performing an initial survey, and evaluating emergency care priorities.

a) *Scene Safety and BSI:* Ensure that you approach the scene safely by checking for potential hazards such as fire, traffic, electrical lines, or environmental concerns. BSI includes wearing appropriate protective gear such as gloves, masks, and eyewear to minimize risk of exposure to bodily fluids.

b) *MOI or NOI:* Determine the cause of injury or illness by gathering information from bystanders or observing surroundings.

c) *AVPU:* Assess mental status using AVPU - Alert, Responsive to Voice or Painful stimuli (Verbal), or Unresponsive.

d) *Initial Survey:* Conduct a rapid visual assessment for life-threatening injuries such as airway obstructions, lack of breathing, severe bleeding, shock symptoms, and chest injuries that impede breathing.

e) *Emergency Care Priorities:* Based on your observations during the initial assessment, determine if immediate life-saving interventions are required before further evaluation.

2. **Secondary Assessment:** Following the primary assessment and any necessary interventions have been performed, proceed to a secondary assessment for a head-to-toe evaluation.

a) *Head:* Examine trauma indicators like skull deformities, wounds, bruises, bruising behind ears (Battle's Sign), and fluid leakage from the ears or nose.

b) *Neck:* Inspect for jugular vein distension, tracheal deviation, neck injuries, or accessory muscle use during breathing.

c) *Chest:* Evaluate the chest for symmetry, deformities such as flail chest, bruising, or open chest wounds.

d) *Abdomen:* Palpate the abdomen for tenderness, rigidity, or distention. Look for signs of injury such as bruises or lacerations.

e) *Pelvis:* Assess for pelvic instability, bruising over the lower region of the back and hips, and localized tenderness.

f) *Extremities:* Examine all limbs for abnormalities such as deformities, swelling, bruising, and open or closed fractures. Check circulation by assessing capillary refill time and distal pulses.

g) *Back:* After spinal immobilization is achieved if indicated, examine the spine for any deformities or injuries.

3. **Triage Process:** Triage is a crucial component of managing multiple patients in mass casualty incidents (MCI). The objective is to prioritize care and allocate resources effectively by categorizing patients based on their injuries' severity.

a) *Immediate (Red):* Severe injuries requiring urgent medical attention that cannot wait until everyone is assessed

b) *Delayed (Yellow):* Patients with non-life-threatening injuries who can wait for treatment but need medical care within a reasonable time

c) *Minor (Green):* Those who have minor injuries that may not require immediate treatment

d) *Deceased/Expectant (Black)*: Individuals who have passed away or have such severe injuries that their chances of survival are negligible even with advanced medical care in providing effective and appropriate prehospital care to patients.

Fractures, Burns, and Soft Tissue Injuries

In this section, we will explore the various types of fractures, burns, and soft tissue injuries that paramedics may encounter during emergency scenarios. An understanding of these injuries is crucial in providing effective and appropriate prehospital care to patients.

1. **Fractures:** Fractures are breaks or disruptions in the continuity of bones. They can result from direct trauma, indirect trauma, or pathological processes. There are several types of fractures that paramedics should be familiar with:

    a) Closed Fracture: The skin over the fracture site remains intact.

    b) Open Fracture: The skin over the fracture site is disrupted, and bone fragments may be visible.

    c) Comminuted Fracture: The bone is broken into multiple fragments.

    d) Spiral Fracture: A twisting force results in a helical fracture line around the bone's axis.

    e) Greenstick Fracture: Only one side of the bone is broken, while the other side remains intact - commonly seen in children.

    f) Pathological Fracture: Caused by a disease process that weakens the bone.

When managing a patient with a suspected fracture, paramedics should obtain a thorough history and perform a systematic physical examination. Pain management is key, along with immobilization of the injured area using splints to prevent further harm and facilitate healing.

2. **Burns:** Burn injuries vary in severity and can result from thermal, chemical, electrical, or radiation exposure. They are classified according to their depth as follows:

    a) First-degree burns: These involve only the epidermis and cause redness and pain without blistering.

    b) Second-degree burns: These extend into the dermis causing blisters and can be superficial (affecting only the upper dermal layer) or deep (affecting deeper dermal layers).

    c) Third-degree burns: These extend through the entire dermis and are characterized by a white, leathery, or charred appearance.

Initial management of burn victims focuses on stopping the burning process, assessing the extent and severity of the burns, and providing appropriate interventions. Fluid resuscitation is crucial for severe burns, and pain management and wound care are essential aspects of treatment.

3. **Soft Tissue Injuries:** Soft tissue injuries encompass injuries to muscles, ligaments,

tendons, fascia, and skin. Some common types of soft tissue injuries include:

a) Lacerations: Cuts or tears in the skin that vary in size, depth, and severity.

b) Contusions: Bruises caused by blunt force trauma that damage underlying tissues without breaking the skin.

c) Abrasions: Superficial injuries where the epidermis is scraped away by friction against a rough surface.

d) Puncture wounds: Deep and usually narrow wounds caused by sharp objects such as nails or needles.

e) Crush injuries: Result from prolonged pressure or compression that damages soft tissues.

Assessment of soft tissue injuries involves identifying any hidden damage, which can be masked by obvious external injuries. Managing soft tissue injuries consists of pain relief measures, wound cleansing/irrigation, bleeding control, dressing application, and immobilization where necessary.

Chapter 8

Life Span Development and Pediatrics

Life Span Development is a crucial aspect of understanding the physiological and psychological transformations that occur at various stages throughout an individual's life. In the field of paramedicine, comprehending these changes is vital when providing care to patients of different age groups, especially in pediatric care.

As a paramedic, recognizing the developmental milestones and knowing how to approach pediatric patients can significantly impact the quality of care provided. A well-rounded understanding of lifespan development will enable paramedics to assess patients accurately, provide appropriate interventions, and communicate effectively.

Let's delve into the significant stages of human development, as they relate to pediatrics:

1. **Neonates (0-28 days):** This stage begins with birth and lasts for approximately one month. It is characterized by rapid growth, intense periods of adjustment for both the neonate and parents, and vulnerability to diseases and infections. In this stage, paramedics should consider factors such as pregnancy history, delivery complications, birthweight, and breathing difficulties when assessing neonates.

2. **Infants (1 month - 1 year):** This period is marked by rapid physical growth and cognitive development. The ability to walk may develop over time, along with increased motor skills, speech acquisition, and social interaction. As paramedics provide care during this stage, they should be aware that infants are susceptible to respiratory issues like bronchiolitis or pneumonia due to their smaller airways.

3. **Toddlers (1-3 years):** During this stage, children experience mobility advancements such

49

as crawling and walking independently. Their cognitive abilities develop further along with language skills improving rapidly. The exploration behavior may lead them to encounter various hazards like choking or accidental poisoning incidents. As a paramedic attending toddlers' emergencies – quick assessment skills; applying PALS guidelines; addressing issues like tantrums or separation anxiety from caregivers is essential.

4. **Preschoolers (3–5 years):** In this age group, children tend to be curious and continue to develop their cognitive and social skills. They can communicate their needs more effectively, making it easier for paramedics to assess during emergencies. When treating preschoolers, paramedics should reassure both the child and the caregiver and provide a prompt yet empathetic clinical service.

5. **School-aged children (6–12 years):** This stage is marked by physical growth, though not as rapid as previous stages; the development of cognitive abilities by experiencing schooling and social skills through interaction with peers and adults. Patients from this age group often benefit from simple explanations of procedures or reassurances that can calm them during emergencies. Paramedics must adapt their communication style to suit school-aged children's knowledge and understanding.

An accurate assessment of pediatric patients requires a modification of usual procedures due to physiological differences in younger patients. When assessing pediatric patients, keep ABCDE (Airway, Breathing, Circulation, Disability, Exposure) principles in mind. The Pediatric Assessment Triangle (PAT) – focusing on appearance, work of breathing, and circulation – is an effective way to gauge the severity of a child's illness or injury rapidly.

Pediatric-specific Considerations

1. **Airway and Breathing:** Children have smaller airways compared to adults and are more prone to obstruction or respiratory distress caused by infections or trauma. Proper positioning, suctioning techniques, oxygen administration and usage of appropriately sized equipment are critical during pediatric airway management.

2. **Circulation:** Pediatric patients have unique circulatory challenges such as faster heart rates and lower blood volumes than adults. It is crucial for paramedics to account for these differences when managing blood pressure or administering medications.

3. **Medication Administration:** Due to their smaller body size and weight, pediatric dosages for medications can differ significantly from adult doses. A thorough understanding of pediatric dosages is vital to avoid adverse effects or inadequate treatments.

4. **Pain Management:** Children may express pain differently than adults, making it challenging to assess their degree of discomfort. Effective pain management in pediatric patients is essential, as it reduces distress and mental trauma during emergencies.

5. **Emotional Care:** Providing emotional care for children and their caregivers during

medical emergencies is paramount. It includes adapting your communication style, utilizing age-appropriate terminologies, and helping them feel at ease.

6.

Chapter 9

Pharmacology and Medication Administration

Among the many responsibilities of a paramedic, understanding pharmacology and medication administration is paramount. This chapter will discuss important aspects related to pharmacology and medication administration, specifically focusing on drug classification and administration routes, as well as calculations and dosages. As a paramedic, mastering this knowledge will enable you to provide safe and effective treatment to your patients.

Drug Classification and Administration Routes

In emergency medicine, paramedics must be familiar with a wide variety of medications used to treat various conditions. Let's discuss drug classification systems and the primary routes of administration used in prehospital care. By understanding these key concepts, paramedics can provide effective medication management for their patients, ensuring they receive the appropriate treatment during emergencies.

Drugs can be classified in several ways based on their chemical structure, pharmacologic effect, and therapeutic use. Understanding drug classifications allows paramedics to anticipate the potential effects of a medication, potential interactions with other drugs, and possible adverse reactions that may occur during administration.

1. **Pharmacologic Classes:** This system organizes drugs based on their pharmacologic effect on the body (i.e., their mechanism of action). Examples include analgesics (pain relief), antipyretics (fever reducers), diuretics (increased urine production), and vasopressors (blood pressure elevation).

2. **Chemical Classes:** Drugs within a chemical class share similar structural features and often have related pharmacologic effects. For example, benzodiazepines are medications with a similar chemical structure that primarily impact the central nervous system to produce sedation, hypnosis, and muscle relaxation.

3. **Therapeutic Classes:** This classification groups drugs based on their therapeutic use or clinical indication. For example, antihypertensive medications lower blood pressure, while bronchodilators relax smooth muscle in the airways to aid in breathing.

There are numerous routes by which drugs can be administered, each with its unique advantages and disadvantages. Becoming proficient in these routes is crucial for paramedics to ensure proper drug delivery in an emergency setting.

1. **Oral (PO):** This is the most common route of administration and involves swallowing the drug, which is then absorbed through the gastrointestinal tract. Oral medications are easy to administer and tend to provide a slower, sustained release of the drug into the bloodstream. However, certain conditions such as vomiting, altered mental status, or head injuries may preclude oral administration.

2. **Intravenous (IV):** This route introduces a drug directly into the bloodstream via a vein, providing rapid onset of action and precise control over dosage. IV administration is commonly used in emergency settings when quick effects are required. However, it also carries risks like infection at the injection site.

3. **Intramuscular (IM):** Drugs administered via intramuscular injection are absorbed more slowly than those given intravenously but still offer a faster onset compared to oral administration. This route is suitable for medications requiring steady absorption into the bloodstream over time.

4. **Subcutaneous (SC or SQ):** Involves injecting the drug into subcutaneous tissue beneath the skin, allowing for slow absorption into the bloodstream. Insulin and various vaccines are often administered subcutaneously and this route is useful when slower absorption is desired.

5. **Inhalation:** Medications can be delivered directly to the respiratory system as aerosols or gases for rapid absorption through lung tissues. This method results in rapid effects as well as minimizing systemic side effects, making inhalation an ideal choice for conditions like asthma or chronic obstructive pulmonary disease (COPD).

6. **Nasal:** Medications can be administered through nasal sprays or drops and rapidly absorbed by mucosal membranes in the nasal cavity, offering quick onset of action.

7. **Rectal:** Although not commonly used in emergency medicine, rectal administration does provide an alternative method for patients unable to tolerate oral medication due in some cases to nausea or unconsciousness.

8. **Topical:** The topical application involves applying a medication directly onto the skin or mucous membranes to achieve local effects. This route is commonly used for treating skin conditions or relieving localized pain and inflammation.

Calculations and Dosages

As a paramedic, you will encounter numerous medications on a regular basis, each requiring specific dosages that are carefully calculated. This process becomes even more complex when the medication is administered intravenously or titrated. Understanding the fundamentals of drug dosage calculations can be the difference between facilitating a smooth recovery for your patient or causing further complications.

When calculating drug dosages, it is essential to remember two basic principles: knowing the desired dosage (as prescribed by a healthcare professional) and understanding the units of measurement. The following measurement systems are commonly used:

a) *Metric System:* commonly used for liquid medications; employing units such as grams, milligrams, micrograms, liters, and milliliters.

b) *Household System:* employs teaspoons, tablespoons, ounces, cups, pints, quarts, etc., although not often used by paramedics.

c) *Apothecary System:* utilizes grains and minims; infrequently used by paramedics.

It's important to know how to convert between these systems when calculating dosages. Familiarize yourself with conversion tables as needed.

Understanding Medication Orders

A physician or medical practitioner often gives medication orders. These orders contain valuable information that enables proper medication calculations and administration:

1. Medication name
2. Dosage form (tablet, liquid, injection)
3. Medication strength
4. Dosage quantity
5. Frequency
6. Route of administration

For example: Morphine Sulfate 10mg IV push q20 minutes prn pain

Basic Medical Math Concepts

Remember the following fundamental medical math conversions for a smooth calculation process:

1. 1 gram (g) = 1,000 milligrams (mg)
2. 1 milligram (mg) = 1,000 micrograms (mcg)
3. 1 kilogram (kg) = 2.2 pounds (lbs)
4. 60 drops per minute (gtts/min) = 1 milliliter per minute (mL/min)

Drug Dosage Calculations

Follow these steps to calculate the appropriate drug dosages:

Step 1: Convert patient weight to kilograms if necessary

Formula: Weight (lbs) / 2.2 = Weight (kg)

Step 2: Determine the ordered dosage using the following formula:

Dosage ordered = Dosage strength × Quantity of drug × Conversion factor

Example: To calculate the required dosage of Amiodarone for a patient weighing 80 kg to have a dose of 5 mg/kg:

80 kg × 5 mg/kg = 400 mg

Infusion Rate Calculations

For medications delivered as a continuous infusion:

Step 1: Determine the total volume of fluid to be infused.

Step 2: Determine the desired time for infusion in hours.

Step 3: Calculate the drop factor (gtts/min)

Formula: Volume (mL)/ Time (hours) × 60 = mL/min

Intravenous (IV) Fluid Calculations

1. Macro drip sets, which deliver large volumes, have a drop factor of 10, 15, or 20 gtts/mL.

2. Micro drip sets, designed for smaller volumes and precise delivery, have a standardized drop factor of 60 gtts/mL.

For IV fluid calculations, use the formula:

Drop factor (gtts/mL) × mL/hour = Drops per minute (gtts/min)

Example: Calculate the IV fluid rate in drops per minute for a patient requiring an infusion rate of 125 mL/hour using a macro drip set with a drop factor of 15 gtts/mL:

15 gtts/mL × 125 mL/hour = 1,875 gtts/hour

1,875 gtts/hour ÷ 60 minutes = approximately 31 gtts/min

Pediatric Drug Dosage Calculation – The Broselow Tape

The Broselow Tape provides an essential reference guide for estimating pediatric dosages safely. Based on weight and age correlations, it categorizes the patient's body surface area and color-codes zones for rapid guidance.

Tips to Avoid Medication Errors

1. Employ the "rights" of medication administration – right patient, right medication, right dose, right route, and right time.
2. Double-check medication names, expiration dates, and doses.
3. Be cautious with calculations involving decimals; remember to add a "leading zero" before decimal points to avoid tenfold dosing errors.
4. Use standardized abbreviations and units of measure.
5. Avoid distractions during medication administration.
6. Communicate with colleagues and healthcare providers regarding medication practices.

Chapter 10

Airway Management and Ventilation

Understanding the strategies and techniques for maintaining open airways, providing adequate oxygenation, and ensuring sufficient ventilation is essential. This chapter serves as an informative guide on the fundamentals of airway management and ventilation for National Registry Paramedic candidates. The following sections will discuss various approaches to airway assessment, techniques for managing airways, mechanical ventilation, oxygen therapy, and common respiratory emergencies.

Airway Assessment and Techniques

The assessment of a patient's airway should be prompt and systematic. Paramedics must first identify any factors that could potentially obstruct the airway, such as foreign bodies, swelling, trauma, fluids, or unconsciousness.

1. **Primary Assessment:** During the primary assessment, consider the patient's presentation, level of consciousness (LOC), and breathing patterns. Inspect the face for signs of distress or trauma by looking for deformities or swelling on or around the mouth, nose, and jaw. Listen for muffled voices, gurgling noises, stridor (high-pitched wheezing sound), snoring respiratory sounds, or inadequate ventilation. These could indicate a partial or complete airway obstruction.

2. **Secondary Assessment:** The secondary assessment delves deeper into the patient's history and involves identifying any underlying medical conditions that may affect their airway management.

A variety of techniques are available to manage an individual's airway in emergencies:

1. **Head-Tilt Chin-Lift:** The head-tilt chin-lift maneuver is a fundamental technique used to open an unresponsive patient's airway quickly. To perform this maneuver:

   a) Place one hand on the patient's forehead and apply gentle pressure.

   b) Place your other hand under the patient's chin and lift it upwards.

   c) Tilt their head backward until the chin is pointing upward.

   This technique moves the tongue away from the back of the throat, reducing the risk of airway obstruction.

2. **Jaw-Thrust Maneuver:** In cases with a possible cervical spine injury, use the jaw-thrust maneuver to avoid causing further damage. To perform this technique:

   a) Kneel at the patient's head, placing your palms against their cheeks.

   b) Place your index and middle finger behind the angle of the jaw and lift it upwards.

   c) Simultaneously move the jaw forward while keeping the head still.

3. **Oropharyngeal Airway (OPA):** An oropharyngeal airway is a plastic device used to maintain an open and unobstructed airway in unconscious patients without a gag reflex. Measure the OPA by aligning it with the patient's earlobe and selecting the correct size. Insert it with the tip facing towards the roof of the mouth, rotating it 180 degrees once you reach the soft palate.

4. **Nasopharyngeal Airway (NPA):** A nasopharyngeal airway is a soft rubber or PVC tube inserted through one nostril to maintain an open airway in conscious or semi-conscious patients. Lubricate the NPA before insertion, measure it by aligning it with the patient's nose and earlobe, and insert it gently at a 90-degree angle into the nostril until reaching the nasopharynx.

5. **Supraglottic Airway Devices:** Supraglottic airway devices, such as laryngeal mask airways (LMA) or King LT airways, are used for passive ventilation in patients at risk of aspiration or when endotracheal intubation is challenging or impossible.

6. **Endotracheal Intubation:** Endotracheal intubation involves inserting a tube directly into the patient's trachea, providing a secure airway and access for mechanical ventilation. This procedure should be performed by well-trained and skilled paramedics, as improper intubation can lead to complications or infections.

Mechanical Ventilation and Oxygen Therapy

Mechanical ventilation and oxygen therapy are essential components of emergency medical services, particularly for paramedics working with critically ill or injured patients. This section will discuss the fundamentals of mechanical ventilation, and important concepts in oxygen therapy for national registry paramedic preparation.

Mechanical Ventilation

Mechanical ventilation refers to the use of a machine or device, such as a ventilator, to assist or replace spontaneous breathing. When considering mechanical ventilation in the EMS setting, it is essential to understand the indications for its use, recognize its potential risks and complications, and have knowledge of various types of ventilator settings.

Indications for mechanical ventilation include respiratory distress that cannot be managed with standard oxygen therapy or non-invasive measures, inability to maintain an adequate airway or protect the airway due to impaired consciousness, apnea, severe hypoxemia despite supplemental oxygen being provided, and severe acidosis resulting from respiratory failure.

The appropriate mode of mechanical ventilation depends on several factors including patient condition and underlying etiology of respiratory failure. Common modes include volume-controlled ventilation (VCV) where a set tidal volume is delivered; pressure-controlled ventilation (PCV) where a set inspiratory pressure is applied; and synchronized intermittent mandatory ventilation (SIMV) where patient-initiated breaths are supported with either pressure support or volume control.

It is imperative that a paramedic closely monitors the patient receiving mechanical ventilation. Common complications include hypoventilation due to inadequate ventilator settings or patient-ventilator dyssynchrony; hyperventilation leading to respiratory alkalosis; barotrauma resulting from excessive pressures being applied; and ventilator-associated pneumonia (VAP). When encountering these complications, it is crucial for paramedics to adjust settings accordingly or contact medical direction for further guidance.

Oxygen Therapy

Oxygen therapy plays an essential role in EMS care by providing supplemental oxygen to patients with decreased oxygen levels or those at risk for hypoxia. The primary goal of oxygen therapy is to maintain adequate tissue oxygenation while minimizing the risk of potential complications such as oxygen toxicity or hypercapnia.

There are various methods for delivering oxygen therapy, including nasal cannulas, simple face masks, non-rebreather masks, and bag-valve-mask devices. Each of these has its own advantages and disadvantages, and paramedics must be skilled in selecting the appropriate method based on their patient's needs.

Nasal cannulas provide low-flow oxygen (1-6 liters/min) and are useful for patients with mild hypoxemia who can maintain their respiratory rate and effort. Simple face masks deliver moderate-flow oxygen (6-10 liters/min) and are an appropriate choice for patients requiring a higher concentration of oxygen than a nasal cannula can provide. Non-rebreather masks can deliver high-flow oxygen (up to 15 liters/min), allowing for a nearly 100% concentration of inspired oxygen which is often necessary in situations such as severe trauma, carbon monoxide poisoning, and severe respiratory distress.

Bag-valve-mask (BVM) devices allow for manual ventilation with supplemental oxygen and can be particularly useful in apneic patients or those with an unprotected airway. When using a BVM device, it is essential to ensure an adequate seal on the patient's face to maximize ventilation efficiency.

Regardless of the method used, it is necessary to continuously monitor the patient's response to therapy. This may include monitoring vital signs such as heart rate, blood pressure, respiratory rate, and pulse oximetry readings; assessing lung sounds; observing skin color; and evaluating mental status changes. Any signs of inadequate response or worsening condition warrant re-assessment of the selected oxygen delivery method and adjustment as necessary.

Respiratory Emergencies

Respiratory emergencies occur when there is an impairment or failure in the respiratory system that leads to insufficient oxygenation or removal of carbon dioxide. Common causes of respiratory emergencies include asthma, chronic obstructive pulmonary disease (COPD), pneumonia, and pulmonary embolism.

Asthma is an inflammatory disease of the airways that leads to bronchoconstriction and mucus production. This restricts airflow and causes wheezing, shortness of breath, and chest tightness. It can be triggered by allergens like pollen, tobacco smoke, or infections. The treatment for asthma attacks involves administering short-acting beta-agonists such as albuterol to relieve bronchospasm; providing oxygen therapy to maintain proper oxygen levels; administering corticosteroids to reduce inflammation; monitoring vital signs; and transporting the patient to the nearest medical facility.

Chronic Obstructive Pulmonary Disease (COPD) is a progressive disease characterized by persistent airflow limitation due to both chronic bronchitis and emphysema. This condition worsens over time and can lead to respiratory failure if not adequately treated. Paramedics can administer supplemental oxygen at 2-4 liters per minute via nasal cannula or non-rebreather mask. The administration of bronchodilators such as albuterol may be beneficial in some cases. Close monitoring of vital signs and rapid transport to a medical facility are essential.

Pneumonia is an infection that causes inflammation within the lungs' air sacs called alveoli. This inflammation leads to fluid accumulation and decreases the ability of the lungs to exchange oxygen and carbon dioxide efficiently. Paramedics can provide supportive treatment with oxygen therapy, monitoring vital signs, and initiating intravenous therapy if necessary. Additional treatments may include bronchodilator administration for wheezing and transporting the patient to a medical facility.

Pulmonary embolism is a life-threatening condition where a blood clot or air bubble blocks one or more pulmonary arteries. This results in decreased blood flow to the lungs, leading to respiratory failure, decreased cardiac output, and shock. The patient may experience chest pain, shortness of breath, tachycardia, hypotension, and possible syncope. The primary management for pulmonary embolism is oxygen administration, monitoring vital signs, initiating intravenous therapy with saline, administering analgesics for pain relief (if prescribed), and rapid transport to a medical facility.

When assessing patients with respiratory emergencies, it is critical to perform a thorough respiratory assessment evaluating the breathing rate, depth, and pattern; breath sounds such as wheezing or crackles which may indicate airway obstruction or secretions; chest movement symmetry; signs of hypoxia including cyanosis (blue skin coloration) or altered mental status; and looking for possible causes of respiratory distress like medical history or environmental factors.

A thorough understanding of respiratory emergencies and their interventions will help you save lives as a paramedic. Familiarize yourself with common presentations of these conditions and learn how to rapidly assess patients in distress. Key components of treating these emergencies include recognizing the underlying cause and providing appropriate support through oxygen therapy, medication administration, and rapid transport to a medical facility.

Chapter 11

Patient Assessment

Patient assessment involves a systematic approach that helps the paramedic to efficiently collect information, identify potential problems, and initiate appropriate interventions. By mastering patient assessment, a paramedic is better equipped to make informed decisions, prioritize care, and provide the highest quality emergency medical service. This chapter will discuss the steps in patient assessment, focusing on the scene size-up and primary assessment as well as the detailed secondary assessment and monitoring.

Scene Size-Up and Primary Assessment

The first step in providing appropriate care is to establish a general understanding of the situation by conducting a scene size-up. This involves a series of steps that help paramedics identify any immediate threats, the number of patients involved, and possible mechanisms of injury.

1. **Ensure scene safety:** Prioritize personal safety and that of your crew. Look for hazards such as downed power lines, leaking gas lines, or aggressive bystanders. Make sure to wear appropriate personal protective equipment (PPE), such as gloves and eye protection, to protect yourself from potential hazards.

2. **Determine mechanism of injury or nature of illness:** Observe the scene for any clues that might indicate the cause of injury or illness. Crash scenes, visible wounds, falls, or seizure-like behavior are examples that can provide vital information on the nature of an incident.

3. **Determine the number of patients:** Establish the number of patients involved in order to determine if additional resources are needed, such as backup ambulance units or specialized teams like hazardous materials team (HAZMAT) or technical rescue team.

4. **Request additional resources if needed:** Once you have identified potential hazards,

assessed mechanism(s) of injury or nature of illness, and determined the number of patients, evaluate whether additional resources are required. Communicate your needs with dispatch in a clear and concise manner.

Upon completion of the scene size-up, it's time to focus on assessing individual patients to determine life-threatening conditions through primary assessment steps.

1. **Form a general impression:** As you approach a patient, assess their general appearance at once. Are they conscious? In distress? Breathing? Are there any signs of immediate life threats, such as severe bleeding or difficulty breathing? This initial impression can help guide your following actions.

2. **Assess mental status using AVPU:** Determine the patient's level of consciousness using the AVPU scale (Alert, Verbal/Painful stimulus, Unresponsive). This provides insight into potential neurological deficits or altered mental status.

3. **Assess airway patency:** Make sure the patient's airway is clear and unrestricted, especially in unconscious patients. An obstructed airway can quickly become life-threatening if not promptly addressed.

4. **Assess breathing:** Verify if the patient is breathing adequately by checking the rate, rhythm and quality of breaths. If a patient is not breathing or has inadequate respirations, provide the appropriate intervention such as rescue breathing or supplemental oxygen.

5. **Assess circulation:** Check for pulse and any obvious signs of external bleeding to ensure proper blood circulation. Rapidly control life-threatening hemorrhages with direct pressure, tourniquets, or hemostatic agents.

6. **Determine transport priority:** Based on your assessment findings, decide whether the patient needs immediate transport or can be further stabilized on-scene before transportation.

Detailed Secondary Assessment

The primary goal of a detailed secondary assessment is to gather specific information about a patient's condition, allowing the paramedic to accurately identify any life-threatening injuries or illnesses. The assessment typically follows a primary survey that checks for immediate threats to life, such as airway obstruction or severe bleeding.

The process of performing a detailed secondary assessment involves several key steps:

1. **Evaluation of Patient History:** Before diving into physical assessments, it's essential to gather relevant information about the patient's past medical history, details about their chief complaint or injury, allergies, medication use, and last oral intake. This can be done using the OPQRSTI-ASPN mnemonic as follows:

   Onset: When did the pain/problem start?

   Provocation: What makes it worse?

Quality: How would you describe your pain/problem?

Radiation: Does the pain radiate anywhere else?

Severity: On a scale from 1 to 10, how severe is your pain/discomfort?

Time: How long have you been experiencing this issue?

Interventions: Have you done anything to try and relieve your symptoms?

- Allergies
- Symptoms
- Past pertinent history
- Last oral intake
- New events related to the current problem

2. **Systematic Head-to-Toe Physical Examination:** A systematic head-to-toe physical examination begins with an assessment of the head and progressively moves down the patient's body, ensuring that all anatomical regions receive thorough attention. This method typically follows these steps:

a) Assess for their level of consciousness and orientation.

b) Examine the head, checking for signs of trauma, deformities, contusions, or lacerations.

c) Inspect the ears for clear fluid (indicating cerebral spinal fluid) or bloody drainage.

d) Evaluate the eyes. Note the pupil size, shape, equality, and reaction to light.

e) Review their airway status, including facial injuries and breathing patterns. Check for any signs of obstructed airways or upper airway compromise.

f) Observe the neck for jugular venous distension (JVD), subcutaneous emphysema, or tracheal deviation using your hands to palpate gently.

g) Inspect the chest, checking for any wounds, bruising, paradoxical movement (flail chest), or impaled objects. Percuss the chest and auscultate lung sounds bilaterally to assess for pneumothorax or hemothorax.

h) Palpate the abdomen for tenderness, guarding, or rigidity, as well as assess for any superficial injuries. If indicated, perform Focused Assessment with Sonography in Trauma (FAST) to look for free intraperitoneal fluid.

i) Evaluate the pelvis by applying gentle pressure to look for signs of instability. Check boxers' area unilaterally by lifting each leg slightly off the ground and giving them a slight shake to differentiate between hip dislocation and pelvic fracture.

j) Assess extremities. Check capillary refill time (CRT), distal pulse strength, motor function/sensation (by asking the patient to wiggle their fingers or toes), and evaluate for injuries such as fractures, dislocations, lacerations/coined injuries/abrasions/contusions/burns/nailbed injuries of fingers and toes.

3. **Vitals Monitoring and Reassessment:** Regularly monitor and record vital signs such as

heart rate, blood pressure, pulse oximetry, respiratory rate, and temperature throughout the assessment to track any changes in the patient's condition. Reassessments should be conducted every 5 minutes for critical patients and every 15 minutes for stable patients to ensure timely detection of any worsening symptoms.

4. **Addressing Life Threats:** During the detailed secondary assessment, it is crucial to remain vigilant about identifying life-threatening conditions that require immediate intervention. This may involve closely monitoring a decreasing Glasgow Coma Scale (GCS) score, sudden decrease in blood pressure, signs of increasing intracranial pressure or shock.

5. **Documenting Findings:** As you conduct your detailed secondary assessment, document all relevant findings in a clear, organized manner that allows other medical professionals to understand your thought process and the care provided to the patient. Record your observations using a standardized format – this will facilitate ease of interpretation by other healthcare providers when printed or accessed electronically.

6. **Communication with Medical Control:** When necessary, request guidance from medical control regarding complex conditions or treatment decisions beyond your scope of practice. Clear communication allows you to receive necessary input while relaying crucial information about your patient's condition accurately.

7. **Patient Care Transfer:** Upon completion of the detailed secondary assessment and any necessary interventions, it is essential to seamlessly transfer your patient's care to the appropriate healthcare provider or facility. During transition, relay your evaluation findings and all provided treatments, ensuring that pertinent details are not lost in translation.

Chapter 12

Special Patient Populations

S pecial patient populations encompass a diverse range of individuals with unique healthcare needs. These groups may require specific assessment and care considerations due to differences in age, physical and psychological conditions, or cultural backgrounds. Paramedics must be aware of these differences and adapt their approach accordingly to provide the best possible care. In this chapter, we will be discussing pediatrics and geriatrics as special patient populations by examining the unique care considerations for both groups.

Pediatrics and Geriatrics Care Considerations

The world of emergency medicine encompasses a wide range of patients, with each group requiring specific attention and care. One area of specialization for paramedics is pediatric and geriatric care. Let's cover some essential considerations that will help you better tailor your approach to these vulnerable populations.

1. Developmental and Physiological Differences in Pediatric Patients: Pediatric patients, defined as those aged 0-18 years old, exhibit numerous differences in anatomy, physiology, and development stages compared to adults. These distinctions significantly impact the assessment and management strategies utilized by paramedics.

Here are a few critical differences to consider:

- *Airway:* A child's airway is shorter than an adult's and may be easily obstructed due to the larger tongue or smaller airway diameter.

- *Breathing:* Infants and young children rely primarily on their diaphragm for breathing, which can fatigue quickly during respiratory distress.

- *Circulation:* Children have faster heart rates compared to adults but lower blood pressure, making it crucial for paramedics to consider signs of shock and compensate accordingly.

- *Head size:* Infants and young children have proportionally larger heads than adults, making them more susceptible to head injuries.

2. Assessment & Management Techniques for Pediatric Patients: When assessing a pediatric patient, expect their reaction to trauma or illness to differ from an adult's. Children may not have the verbal skills to communicate their symptoms or may be unable to cooperate due to fear.

In these cases, use the following approaches:

- Remain calm and approach the child gently; build trust before examination
- Use objective assessment tools like the Pediatric Assessment Triangle or Apgar Score
- Adjust vital sign reference values based on age
- Exercise extreme caution when immobilizing the spine; use appropriately-sized cervical collars

3. Developmental & Physiological Changes in Geriatric Patients: Geriatric patients, typically defined as those over 65 years old, require unique care considerations due to their physical and cognitive changes.

Here are a few key differences to consider:

- *Cardiovascular:* With age, the heart becomes less efficient in pumping blood, and blood vessels lose elasticity. This leads to a reduced ability to tolerate stressors such as dehydration or blood loss.
- *Respiratory:* Lung function decreases with age, reducing oxygen exchange capacity and making older adults more susceptible to respiratory illnesses.
- *Cognitive:* Aging can result in cognitive decline, potentially making assessment and communication with geriatric patients more challenging.
- *Polypharmacy:* Geriatric patients often have multiple medical conditions that are treated with numerous medications that may interact or contribute to emergency situations.

4. Assessment & Management Techniques for Geriatric Patients: Geriatric emergencies often present atypically or develop complications that require targeted assessment techniques:

- Utilize a systematic but patient-specific approach; consider and rule out diagnoses with high morbidity or mortality
- Develop rapport by addressing elderly patients respectfully and using their preferred name
- Be cautious when immobilizing the spine since older adults may have pre-existing spinal conditions that make immobilization contraindicated
- Ask about medications taken regularly or recently ceased; these may aid in understanding underlying causes of the emergency

5. Special Considerations for Both Populations: Certain situations arise in both pediatric and geriatric populations that necessitate specialized recognition and intervention:

— *Falls:* Both groups are at an increased risk of falls; attention should be given to injury prevention measures to reduce fall-related morbidity.

— *End-of-life care:* Paramedics must provide culturally sensitive care within the bounds of their scope of practice while considering family decisions (e.g., do not resuscitate orders) during end-of-life situations.

— *Mental health:* Be aware of psychiatric illnesses that can manifest physical symptoms or exacerbate underlying medical conditions.

Chapter 13

EMS Operations and Incident Command

E MS Operations encompass the principles, practices, and procedures required for the safe and efficient delivery of medical care during emergencies. In contrast, Incident Command refers to a structured system that establishes a chain of command and aims to coordinate efforts, allocate resources, and streamline communication within multiple agencies responding to any mass casualty incidents (MCI). This chapter will provide an overview of essential EMS Operations concepts such as ambulance operations and safety, along with an understanding of the Incident Command System when managing mass casualty incidents.

Ambulance Operations and Safety

As first responders, paramedics must not only have the skills and knowledge to save lives but also operate ambulances safely and efficiently. The first aspect of ambulance operations is the vehicle's overall design. Several factors contribute to an ambulance's design, including meeting the needs of individual EMS agencies and complying with national standards. The most common ambulance types are Type I, Type II, and Type III, which differ by chassis type and specifications.

In all ambulances, lighting is integral to ensuring visibility for safe driving during both day and nighttime operations. Emergency lights consist of red, blue, white, or amber flashing lights that alert the public to the presence of an emergency vehicle. Additionally, headlamps provide illumination during nighttime hours for easy identification. The siren system functions to warn nearby motorists when an ambulance approaches intersections or operates at high speeds.

Vehicle maintenance is another critical aspect of ambulance operation. Paramedics must ensure that their ambulance is in proper working order through regular inspections, which include checking fluid levels and tire pressure. Keeping emergency equipment clean, organized, and accessible will also contribute to smooth operations during emergencies.

Driving techniques play a vital role in maintaining safety during response and transport. Paramedics must successfully navigate through traffic with minimal risk while adhering to traffic laws. This requires staying vigilant while scanning the road ahead for potential hazards like roadblocks or pedestrians crossing unexpectedly.

In addition to driving safely on open roads, paramedics must master response codes tied explicitly to each emergency call. These codes range from 'no lights or sirens' (Code 1) all the way up to 'lights and sirens at maximum capacity' (Code 3). By adhering to these codes, paramedics minimize the risk of accidents while responding to calls and maintain public safety always.

The principle of "due regard" is a cornerstone of ambulance operations, and it is the legal responsibility paramedics have when operating emergency vehicles. Paramedics must drive with due care and caution, which includes adjusting their driving behavior according to weather conditions, traffic situations, or road hazards. They must also consider other drivers' reactions when driving with emergency lights and sirens, as the sudden presence of an emergency vehicle can lead to confusion or panic.

During patient transport, several measures ensure a high level of safety for both patients and paramedics. One such measure is securing the patient safely using straps and restraints to prevent movement during transport. Another essential aspect is communicating effectively with other crew members regarding any changes in the patient's medical condition or additional assistance needed.

Transportation that prioritizes patient safety is essential in ambulance operations. Many factors come into play, such as driving at controlled speeds to minimize unnecessary movement within the vehicle or choosing routes that avoid bumpy roads or excessive turns. Furthermore, the driver should make regular updates on their estimated time of arrival (ETA) to the receiving hospital so that staff can be ready upon their arrival.

Paramedics must consider patient comfort during transport as well. This involves adjusting temperature controls within the ambulance to maintain a suitable environment for those inside, taking care not to exacerbate any injuries or illnesses. Moreover, practitioners should inform their patients about any sudden movements or turns made during transportation to minimize stress or anxiety.

Incident Command System and Mass Casualty Incidents

In emergency situations, rapid and efficient response coordination is essential to maximize the chances of success. One of the key tools in a first responder's toolkit is the Incident Command System (ICS), which provides a standardized and flexible approach to managing complex incidents.

The Incident Command System is a proven framework that is scalable, adaptable, and applicable to all hazardous emergencies or non-emergency incidents. The ICS aims to provide efficient communication channels and coordination methods during emergency response operations, including those that involve multiple agencies or jurisdictions.

One significant aspect of the ICS is its organizational structure, which consists of five primary functional areas: Command, Operations, Planning, Logistics, and Finance/Administration.

1. **Command:** The primary decision-making authority in charge of the entire incident response. The Incident Commander (IC) provides strategic guidance and sets objectives for response efforts.

2. **Operations:** This section focuses on direct tactical actions and resource allocation required for managing the incident. It includes personnel placement, task assignment, and incident stabilization efforts.

3. **Planning:** The Planning Section gathers information relevant to the incident, develops action plans, analyzes data while monitoring ongoing operations, and revises plans as needed.

4. **Logistics:** This section is responsible for providing material support such as equipment, supplies, facilities, transportation services, and personnel required by other sections.

5. **Finance/Administration:** The Finance/Administration Section addresses financial aspects such as cost analysis documentation, procurement processes, compensation claims handling situations involving injured responders or damaged properties.

In a mass casualty incident (MCI), there are typically numerous victims involved with varying degrees of injuries requiring immediate medical attention. MCIs can quickly exceed local resources' capacity in terms of personnel or medical supply demands; this makes an effective situation management crucial for saving lives. The ICS can be invaluable in coordinating response efforts during such incidents.

When an MCI occurs, the IC must quickly establish a unified command system to enable seamless communication and collaboration among all involved agencies. The IC identifies critical objectives and sets priorities based on the severity of injuries, available resources, and potential for further danger. This prioritization helps ensure that the most urgent cases are treated first.

Next, the IC assigns tasks to the appropriate sections within the ICS framework. For example, the Operations Section would deploy emergency medical services (EMS) personnel to triage, treat, and transport patients. The Logistics Section gathers crucial medical supplies and equipment for resource allocation to aid in providing care for victims.

The Planning Section plays an important role in analyzing data, employing MCI-specific guidelines in coordination with other involved parties such as hospitals condition reports and their capacity to treat more patients.

During an MCI, one challenge is triaging patients effectively based on their injury severity.

Triage is vital to ensuring that scarce resources are allocated according to need. Various triage systems can be utilized during MCIs, such as the START (Simple Triage and Rapid Treatment) or JumpSTART systems for pediatric patients.

Once triage has been completed, EMS personnel provide initial treatment to stabilize patients to the best of their capability within resource constraints. These treatments may include basic life support (BLS), advanced life support (ALS), or other minimal interventions.

Another essential aspect of managing an MCI is patient transportation and appropriate destination selection based on facility capability and load balance considerations. Evacuation plans should be well-coordinated with designated receiving facilities under close communication with them. Plans should also account for intra-hospital patient transfers once they've been admitted.

MCIs are chaotic situations that test a community's preparedness level and response capabilities; they require rapid adaptation and clear decision making under intense pressure. ICS provides a proven management framework assisting in coordinating, controlling, and communicating throughout the response to these challenging events.

Chapter 14

Medical Legal and Ethical Considerations

When working in the field of emergency medical services, paramedics are required to navigate the complex web of medical legalities and ethical considerations. This chapter presents important information on the legal, ethical, and professional responsibilities of a paramedic when interacting with patients. National Registry Paramedic candidates must comprehend and adhere to these guidelines to ensure they are providing the highest level of patient care while protecting patient rights and their own professional standing.

Consent, Documentation, and HIPAA

In this section, we will delve into the critical concepts surrounding consent, documentation, and compliance with the Health Insurance Portability and Accountability Act (HIPAA) within the scope of paramedic practice.

Consent

Obtaining informed consent from patients or their legal guardians is a crucial aspect of paramedic practice. When attending to an emergency or providing care, paramedics need to ensure that the patients understand the necessity for treatment as well as the potential risks and benefits involved.

Informed consent is defined as the patient's voluntary agreement to undergo a particular medical procedure or accept care after receiving a comprehensive explanation of risks, benefits, and alternatives. To establish informed consent, paramedics must:

- Provide accurate information about treatments or procedures in easily understandable terms
- Confirm patient understanding
- Ensure that the patient voluntarily agrees to the suggested course of action.

There are three main types of consent:

a) *Express consent:* This type of consent can be obtained verbally or in writing when a conscious patient clearly communicates their willingness to receive care.

b) *Implied consent:* Implied consent refers to situations where a patient is unconscious, unable to communicate, or lacks decision-making capacity, but it is reasonable to assume that they would want help if they could communicate appropriately. This type of consent typically applies in emergency situations.

c) *Consent for minors:* Legally, children (under 18) cannot provide their own consent; thus, parents or legal guardians must provide permission on their behalf. Exceptions to this rule include emancipated minors and instances where obtaining guardian consent would delay life-saving treatment.

Documentation

Documentation by paramedics plays a vital role in supporting continuity of care for patients while also serving as a crucial communication tool for healthcare teams. The primary documentation tool used by paramedics is the Patient Care Report (PCR). It records patient assessment findings, vital signs, interventions, and other relevant data.

Some essential elements of the PCR include:

a) *Demographic information:* Patient demographics, incident location, and transport destination.

b) *Chief complaint:* Primary reason for requesting medical assistance in the patient's own words if available.

c) *Medical history, medications, and allergies*

d) *Detailed assessment findings:* Systematic physical examination and vital signs recorded at different stages of care (initial assessment and ongoing re-assessment).

e) *Treatment provided:* Medical interventions performed by the paramedics and associated results or patient responses.

f) *Narrative summary:* A comprehensive account of patient interaction in chronological order.

Paramedics must provide accurate, timely, and complete documentation to ensure the following:

- Compliance with legal requirements
- Communication with subsequent medical providers
- Protection against potential litigation

Inaccurate or incomplete documentation can jeopardize patient care, leading to potential malpractice lawsuits and losing EMS licenses.

HIPAA Compliance

Under the Health Insurance Portability and Accountability Act (HIPAA), paramedics must adhere to specific guidelines that regulate healthcare information privacy and security. HIPAA stipulates several key principles that aim to safeguard personal health information (PHI). Some fundamental aspects for paramedics include:

a) Obtain signed PHI release forms before sharing patient information with non-healthcare entities.

b) Only exchange necessary PHI when discussing patient care.

c) Safeguard physical copies of PCRs from unauthorized access.

d) Implement strong passwords for logging onto electronic devices containing PHI.

e) Regularly update antivirus software on laptops storing PHI.

Breaches occur when unauthorized individuals gain access to PHI or use it inappropriately. If a breach is detected, paramedics must notify their supervisor and follow the appropriate protocol.

Legal and Ethical Dilemmas in Paramedic Practice

In the dynamic environment of modern healthcare, it is imperative that paramedics are aware of the legal and ethical dilemmas they may confront during their practice. This section aims to provide an overview of some common legal and ethical dilemmas and discusses strategies for addressing these challenges.

1. **Consent and Decision-Making Capacity:** One of the most frequently encountered legal dilemmas for paramedics is obtaining informed consent from the patient before initiating treatment. Informed consent requires that patients are provided with accurate information about the risks, benefits, and alternatives for every intervention and must be obtained before initiating treatment, whenever possible.

   The decision-making capacity of patients can be incredibly complex, especially when dealing with trauma or behavioral health issues. A patient may also be under the influence of drugs or alcohol, exacerbating the dilemma. In such situations, it is crucial for paramedics to exercise professional judgment in determining if a patient has the capacity to give informed consent.

2. **End-of-Life Care and DNR Orders:** Fulfilling end-of-life care wishes can present ethical challenges for paramedics when faced with Do-Not-Resuscitate (DNR) orders or Advance Directives. In these instances, a paramedic may encounter a situation where they must choose between honoring a patient's preferences and performing life-saving interventions.

   It is important to remember that honoring the wishes of a patient is an essential aspect of providing compassionate care. However, encountering unclear or ambiguous directives can lead to confusion as to how to proceed. When in doubt, consulting with medical control can provide guidance on interpreting such orders.

3. **Confidentiality and Patient Privacy:** Paramedics face constant legal and ethical challenges related to confidentiality and patient privacy concerns. During prehospital care, they must balance the need to share critical information with colleagues and emergency departments, while maintaining the privacy of patients according to Health Insurance Portability and Accountability Act (HIPAA) rules. Paramedics should strive to exercise caution, disclosing only essential information required for appropriate patient care. Any breach in patient confidentiality can expose paramedics to legal and professional difficulties.

4. **Treatment of Minors:** When treating minors, the consent of a parent or legal guardian is typically required before treatment. However, during emergencies or when a guardian is not present at the scene, obtaining consent can be challenging. In these cases, it may be necessary for paramedics to treat the minor under the implied consent doctrine, assuming that a reasonable guardian would consent to treatment under the circumstances.

5. **Mandatory Reporting:** Paramedics are sometimes faced with ethical dilemmas regarding mandatory reporting situations, such as when witnessing child abuse or neglect. This task can be particularly difficult as it may involve reporting suspicions about people whom they have built rapport with in their community.
In such cases, paramedics have a legal obligation to report instances of abuse or neglect and should follow local laws and protocols for doing so. It is essential to understand that the primary goal of reporting is to protect vulnerable individuals from harm and not intended as punitive measures against those suspected of wrongdoing.

6. **Resource Management:** Situations where resources are limited can pose significant ethical challenges for paramedics as they struggle to provide adequate care for multiple patients simultaneously. Making tough decisions under high-pressure scenarios is what paramedics are trained for but can undoubtedly weigh heavily on them emotionally.
In moments like these, it is crucial to remember that strict prioritization based on patient severity can help alleviate some decision-making burden. Utilizing resources such as mass casualty algorithms can also help guide paramedics in determining which patients need attention most urgently.

Chapter 15

Practice Exams and Answers

I. General Knowledge And Skills

1. What is the primary function of the respiratory system?

   a) To transport oxygen and nutrients

   b) To provide structural support for the body

   c) To exchange gases between the body and the environment

   d) To transmit sensory information

2. Which blood vessel carries oxygen-rich blood from the lungs to the heart?

   a) Aorta

   b) Pulmonary artery

   c) Pulmonary vein

   d) Vena cava

3. Which part of a neuron receives messages from other neurons?

   a) Axon

   b) Dendrite

   c) Cell body

   d) Myelin sheath

4. What type of joint allows for movement in all directions?

   a) Hinge joint

   b) Ball-and-socket joint

   c) Pivot joint

d) Gliding joint

5. Which hormone regulates blood sugar levels?

a) Insulin
b) Cortisol
c) Adrenaline
d) Oxytocin

6. How many lobes are present in the right lung?

a) 2
b) 3
c) 4
d) 5

7. What is the largest artery in the body?

a) Aorta
b) Carotid artery
c) Femoral artery
d) Vena cava

8. Which division of the nervous system controls involuntary functions?

a) Central nervous system
b) Peripheral nervous system
c) Autonomic nervous system
d) Somatic nervous system

9. Which type of muscle is found in the walls of internal organs and blood vessels?

a) Skeletal muscle
b) Smooth muscle
c) Cardiac muscle
d) Connective tissue

10. Which gland is responsible for producing the hormone thyroxine, which regulates metabolism?

a) Adrenal gland
b) Pituitary gland
c) Pineal gland
d) Thyroid gland

11. Which of the following refers to "pain in a joint"?

a) Arthropathy

b) Arthritis

c) Arthralgia

d) Myalgia

12. What does the term "dyspnea" mean?

a) Rapid breathing

b) Irregular breathing

c) Difficulty breathing

d) Shallow breathing

13. What does the term "hypoxia" refer to?

a) High blood pressure

b) Low blood sugar levels

c) Decreased oxygen in the body

d) Increased carbon dioxide in the body

14. What does the term "tachycardia" refer to?

a) A slow heart rate

b) A rapid heart rate

c) An irregular heart rate

d) A normal heart rate

15. The suffix "-itis" commonly refers to:

a) Swelling

b) Inflammation

c) Pain

d) Abnormal growth

16. Which of the following best describes the primary cause of systemic inflammation in sepsis?

a) Release of endotoxins by bacteria

b) Overproduction of white blood cells

c) Hypoxia due to ineffective tissue perfusion

d) The body's inability to maintain homeostasis

17. In a patient suffering from congestive heart failure, which pathophysiologic mechanism commonly causes pulmonary edema?

a) Increased preload

b) Increased afterload

c) Decreased cardiac contractility

d) Decreased systemic vascular resistance

18. The primary reason for hypoperfusion in anaphylactic shock is due to:

    a) Massive vasodilation

    b) Direct myocardial depression

    c) Significant fluid loss into the interstitial space

    d) Systemic vasoconstriction leading to tissue ischemia

19. How does pathophysiology of tension pneumothorax mainly affect the cardiovascular system?

    a) Compression of the heart and great vessels, impeding venous return and cardiac output

    b) Necrosis of myocardial tissue due to obstruction of coronary arteries

    c) Decreased stroke volume and cardiac output caused by pericardial tamponade

    d) Systemic arterial and venous vasodilation, reducing peripheral resistance

20. In a patient with Type 1 diabetes, what is the primary cause for diabetic ketoacidosis (DKA)?

    a) Excessive insulin administration

    b) Severe dehydration caused by elevated blood glucose levels

    c) Lack of insulin leading to the breakdown of fats for energy and increased ketone production

    d) Elevated production of glucagon stimulating glycogenolysis

II. Patient Assessment And Clinical Decision Making

21. Which of the following steps should be taken first in a scene size-up?

    a) Assessing the mechanism of injury/nature of illness

    b) Identifying the number of patients

    c) Ensuring scene safety

    d) Donning personal protective equipment

22. What is the primary reason for using personal protective equipment (PPE) during a call?

    a) To maintain professionalism

    b) To protect the patient from infection

    c) To protect the paramedic from hazards and contaminants

    d) To comply with local regulations

23. When determining the number of patients at a scene, what should a paramedic take into account?

    a) Only patients requiring immediate treatment

    b) Only patients requiring Advanced Life Support (ALS) intervention

    c) All individuals involved, regardless of injury severity

d) Only patients found within 25 feet of an incident

24. Which is NOT considered part of the mechanism of injury assessment during a scene size-up?

a) Evaluating environmental factors that may pose additional risks to yourself or patient
b) Recognizing potential violence or danger at a crime scene
c) Style and make of the vehicles involved in an accident
d) Media review on what happened

25. During your Scene Size-Up when determining the nature of illness, which source will provide you valuable information about your patient's condition?

a) Dispatch Information/Updates
b) Patient's Family or Friends
c) On-scene signs and symptoms
d) All the above

26. Which of the following is NOT a component of a general impression during the Primary Assessment?

a) Appearance of the patient
b) Body posture
c) Verbal responsiveness
d) Past medical history

27. During Airway, Breathing, and Circulation (ABC) assessment, what is the first step in managing a patient's airway?

a) Insertion of a nasopharyngeal airway
b) Application of high-flow oxygen via a non-rebreather mask
c) Opening the airway using head-tilt chin-lift or jaw-thrust maneuver
d) Auscultation of breath sounds

28. When assessing circulation in the Primary Assessment, which of the following should be evaluated first?

a) Blood pressure
b) Skin color, temperature, and condition
c) Pulse rate and quality
d) Capillary refill time

29. Which method should be used to open the airway in a patient with suspected spinal injury during Primary Assessment?

a) Head-tilt chin-lift maneuver
b) Jaw-thrust maneuver without head extension

c) Oropharyngeal airway insertion

d) Finger sweep technique

30. In a Primary Assessment, which part of body structure evaluation involves checking for deformities, contusions, abrasions, punctures, penetrations, burns, and tenderness?

a) Palpation

b) Percussion

c) Auscultation

d) Inspection

31. During a secondary assessment, which of the following vital signs is NOT typically monitored?

a) Heart rate

b) Blood pressure

c) Respiratory rate

d) Height

32. During a head-to-toe examination, upon examining the patient's chest, which of the following conditions might be suspected if the patient has diminished and unequal breath sounds?

a) Asthma

b) Pneumothorax

c) Chronic bronchitis

d) Pulmonary embolism

33. What does the acronym "SAMPLE" stand for in history taking?

a) Signs/Symptoms, Allergies, Medications, Past medical history, Last oral intake, Events leading to present illness/injury

b) Severity, Associated symptoms, Medications, Prior medical history, Last meal, Exacerbating/Relieving factors

c) Severity, Airways, Musculoskeletal issues, Past conditions, Location of pain/injury, Environment surrounding incident

d) Signs/Symptoms, Associated risks, Major concerns, Present health status, Likely cause of injury/illness, Emergency response needed

34. Which of the following measurements is NOT commonly assessed during a secondary exam focused on vital signs?

a) Pulse oximetry

b) Pain scale rating

c) Capillary refill time

d) Glucose level

35. When performing a head-to-toe examination on a trauma patient with a suspected spinal injury while maintaining spinal precautions as required by NREMT protocols for paramedics – what should you do FIRST after assessing airway and breathing status?

   a) Assess pupillary response
   b) Log roll the patient for back and spine examination
   c) Apply a cervical collar
   d) Assess sensation and motor function in extremities

36. A 45-year-old female presents with chest pain and difficulty breathing. Her vital signs are BP 150/90, HR 110, RR 22, SpO2 92% on room air. Which of the following should be your initial intervention?

   a) Administer nitroglycerin
   b) Perform a 12-lead ECG
   c) Apply high-flow oxygen via non-rebreather mask
   d) Initiate rapid sequence intubation

37. A pediatric patient presents with symptoms of anaphylaxis, including respiratory distress and widespread hives after ingesting peanuts. Which of the following medications should you prioritize for administration?

   a) Epinephrine
   b) Diphenhydramine (Benadryl)
   c) Albuterol
   d) Furosemide (Lasix)

38. In which of the following situations would you most likely administer intraosseous (IO) access in a pediatric patient who needs intravenous (IV) medication administration?

   a) Mild dehydration due to gastroenteritis
   b) Seizure lasting longer than 5 minutes
   c) Cardiac arrest with persistent bradycardia
   d) Closed radius fracture needing pain management

39. An unresponsive elderly patient has been found lying on the floor of their bedroom without any obvious injuries including no trauma nor bleeding, and there is no indication of how long they have been down. Concerning her Advanced Life Support (ALS) interventions, what would be your first step in assessing this patient's condition and formulating an appropriate course of action?

   a) Attach AED to check for shockable rhythm/arrhythmia
   b) Establish an IV line for rapid fluid administration
   c) Apply a cervical collar and secure to a backboard
   d) Perform a primary rapid trauma assessment starting with airway evaluation

40. **A male patient has sustained a penetrating gunshot wound to the right side of his chest. He presents with absent breath sounds on the right side, tracheal deviation, and increasing respiratory distress. Optimal management of this injury initially should consist of:**

   a) Chest decompression using a needle thoracostomy
   b) Application of an occlusive chest seal
   c) Administration of high-flow oxygen via non-rebreather mask
   d) Initiation of rapid sequence intubation (RSI)

III. Medical Emergencies

41. **Which of the following is not a common sign of Acute Coronary Syndrome (ACS)?**

   a) Chest pain
   b) Shortness of breath
   c) Nausea
   d) Joint stiffness

42. **What is the first-line treatment for ventricular fibrillation in an arrhythmia management scenario?**

   a) Amiodarone administration
   b) Defibrillation
   c) Lidocaine administration
   d) Cardiopulmonary resuscitation (CPR)

43. **Which medication is commonly used as a bronchodilator in the treatment of asthma exacerbation?**

   a) Epinephrine
   b) Albuterol
   c) Dexamethasone
   d) Aspirin

44. **What is the primary cause of Chronic Obstructive Pulmonary Disease (COPD)?**

   a) Smoking
   b) Allergies
   c) Air pollution
   d) Obesity

45. **Which type of seizure is characterized by a sudden loss of muscle tone and a brief loss of consciousness?**

   a) Absence seizure
   b) Complex partial seizure

c) Atonic seizure

d) Tonic-clonic seizure

46. The acronym FAST is used primarily for stroke assessment and stands for:

a) Frowning, Arm drift, Slurred speech, Time to call for help.

b) Face drooping, Arm weakness, Speech difficulty, Time to call 911.

c) Facial asymmetry, Arm drift, Slurred speech, Timely intervention.

d) Face weakness, Arm paralysis, Speech problems, Time to call EMS.

47. A patient with gastrointestinal bleeding is exhibiting signs of hypovolemic shock. What is the main priority for this patient's management?

a) Improving oxygenation

b) Stopping the bleeding

c) Providing antiemetics

d) Aggressive fluid resuscitation

48. Diabetic Ketoacidosis (DKA) is an endocrine emergency most commonly found in patients with:

a) Type 1 diabetes

b) Type 2 diabetes

c) Hypothyroidism

d) Hyperthyroidism

49. Which of the following treatments is not recommended during an anaphylactic allergic reaction?

a) Administering epinephrine

b) Administering intravenous fluids

c) Administering a saline nebulizer treatment

d) Administering an antihistamine medication

50. Priority treatment for patients exposed to carbon monoxide poisoning includes:

a) Obtaining a blood sugar level.

b) Administration of supplemental oxygen.

c) Inducing vomiting.

d) Gastric lavage.

IV. Trauma Care

51. What is the primary method of controlling external bleeding in a trauma patient?

a) Direct pressure

b) Tourniquet placement

c) Elevation
d) Cold application

52. In a trauma patient with suspected hypovolemic shock, what is the first-line treatment approach?

a) Administer high-flow oxygen
b) Initiate cold therapy
c) Apply direct pressure to bleeding sites
d) Administer IV fluids

53. Which of the following is an essential consideration in the initial management of burn injuries?

a) Removing all clothing surrounding the burn
b) Rapid cooling of the burn site with ice
c) Initiating fluid administration immediately
d) Stopping the burning process by flushing with water

54. When assessing a patient with suspected spinal injury, what is the primary goal of spinal immobilization?

a) Reduction of pain and discomfort
b) Prevention of spinal curvature
c) Prevention of secondary injury due to movement
d) Promotion of proper posture and alignment

55. In a burn injury, which depth classification involves damage to all layers of skin and underlying structures?

a) Superficial burns
b) Partial-thickness burns
c) Full-thickness burns
d) Immersion burns

56. What is one major contraindication for using a tourniquet in bleeding control?

a) Fractured extremity
b) Arterial bleeding at the extremity
c) Venous bleeding at the extremity
d) Junctional hemorrhage

57. Which type of shock results from trauma-induced fluid loss?

a) Hypovolemic shock
b) Cardiogenic shock
c) Septic shock

d) Neurogenic shock

58. When should a paramedic use a cervical collar for spinal immobilization?

a) The patient has unresponsive muscles in the extremities
b) The patient has midline neck tenderness
c) The patient has a history of chronic neck pain
d) The patient complains of a headache

59. Which of the following extrication devices is designed for rapid removal of patients from motor vehicle accidents?

a) KED (Kendrick Extrication Device)
b) Scoop stretcher
c) Pediatric immobilization device
d) Long spine board

60. Which factor is essential to consider when estimating the severity of burns in a trauma patient?

a) Percentage of body surface area affected
b) The thickness of the skin around the burn
c) The initial temperature of the burning agent
d) The color and appearance of burn wounds

V. Pediatric Care

61. What is the first step in assessing a pediatric patient in an emergency situation?

a) Obtain a medical history
b) Perform a physical exam
c) Check for signs of distress
d) Evaluate their airway, breathing, and circulation (ABCs)

62. In the Pediatric Assessment Triangle (PAT), what components are assessed?

a) Appearance, work of breathing, and circulation to the skin
b) Airway, breathing, and circulation
c) Heart rate, respiratory rate, and mental status
d) Capillary refill time, blood pressure, and oxygen saturation

63. What is the appropriate compression-to-ventilation ratio for single-rescuer infant CPR?

a) 15:2
b) 30:2
c) 5:1
d) 10:1

64. In pediatric resuscitation, why is it important to avoid over-ventilating the patient?

    a) This can impair venous return to the heart and reduce cerebral blood flow.

    b) It may cause oxygen toxicity.

    c) It can dangerously increase intracranial pressure.

    d) It may lead to hypoxia.

65. What is the recommended fluid bolus for a pediatric patient in shock?

    a) 20 mL/kg

    b) 10 mL/kg

    c) 5 mL/kg

    d) 30 mL/kg

66. Which of the following is not included in assessing signs of distress in pediatrics?

    a) ABCs and level of consciousness

    b) Stridor or wheezing sounds while inhaling or exhaling

    c) Cyanosis or pallor of skin color

    d) Minimum weight-bearing ability

67. Which technique could be used when managing potential pediatric foreign body airway obstruction for infants under one year old?

    a) J-thrust

    b) Back blows and chest thrusts

    c) Chin-lift, head-tilt maneuver

    d) Abdominal thrusts (Heimlich maneuver)

68. In pediatric resuscitation, what is the recommended defibrillator dose for an automated external defibrillator (AED)?

    a) 2 Joules/kg

    b) 5 Joules/kg

    c) 4 Joules/kg

    d) Adult-dose pads but with a pediatric attenuator

69. Which medication can be used for pediatric cardiac arrest with pulseless ventricular tachycardia or ventricular fibrillation?

    a) Lidocaine

    b) Adenosine

    c) Epinephrine

    d) Amiodarone

70. What is the age range generally considered to be pediatric in emergency care?

    a) Birth to 8 years old

b) Birth to 12 years old
c) Birth to 18 years old
d) Birth to 21 years old

VI. Obstetrics And Gynecological Emergencies

71. Which of the following is NOT a sign of imminent childbirth?

a) Contractions less than two minutes apart
b) Dilated cervix
c) Crowning
d) Fluid-filled silicone breast implant rupture

72. Breech presentation is when the:

a) Head presents first
b) Buttocks or feet present first
c) Umbilical cord presents first
d) Placenta presents first

73. Shoulder dystocia is a complication in which:

a) The baby's head emerges but the shoulders get stuck behind the pelvic bone
b) The baby's shoulders emerge before the head
c) The umbilical cord is wrapped around the baby's neck or body
d) The pregnant individual experiences severe abdominal pain during labor

74. In a normal delivery, which fetal position is considered most ideal?

a) Vertex, occiput anterior
b) Vertex, occiput posterior
c) Breech, frank position
d) Breech, complete position

75. A prolapsed umbilical cord is considered an emergency situation because:

a) It can cause infection in the newborn
b) It can lead to a prolonged Labor and Delivery process
c) It can cause oxygen deprivation and bradycardia in the newborn if not corrected promptly
d) It usually indicates that there is also a nuchal cord present

76. When providing an emergency childbirth assistance, which stage of labor ends with the expulsion of the placenta?

a) First stage of labor
b) Second stage of labor
c) Third stage of labor

d) Fourth stage of labor

77. During an urgent childbirth situation, what must be done immediately after the baby's head emerges?

a) Clearing airway, ensuring there is no cord around the neck
b) Checking fetal heart rate
c) Wiping all meconium from the baby's face
d) Applying a sterile dressing over the baby's head

78. A newborn presented with APGAR scores of 1, 1, and 2 in Appearance, Pulse, and Grimace, respectively. What is the total APGAR score?

a) 3
b) 4
c) 5
d) 6

79. In case of a precipitous delivery, what position should you place the pregnant individual?

a) Left lateral recumbent position
b) Supine with a foot elevated
c) Semi-Fowler's position
d) On their back with knees bent or slightly modified lithotomy position

80. For a postpartum hemorrhage related to uterine atony, which of the following would be an appropriate first-line intervention?

a) Fundal massage
b) IV fluids (crystalloids)
c) Administration of uterotonic agents (Oxytocin)
d) Blood transfusion

VII. Special Patient Populations

81. Which of the following is commonly observed in geriatric patients with a hip fracture?

a) Bruising on the abdomen
b) Shortened and externally rotated leg
c) Swollen knee joint
d) Numbness in the foot

82. When interacting with a patient with a hearing disability, which approach is most appropriate for effective communication?

a) Speak louder and slower
b) Use written communication if possible

c) Ignore the disability and speak normally

d) Ask the patient to read your lips

83. In geriatric patients, which of these respiratory issues may be more prevalent due to decreased lung elasticity?

a) Asthma

b) Pneumonia

c) Bronchitis

d) Emphysema

84. When assessing a patient with an intellectual disability, it is important to:

a) Rush the assessment to avoid causing anxiety

b) Speak only to the caregiver for medical information

c) Use simple language and ask one question at a time

d) Assume the patient cannot understand you and avoid direct communication

85. Geriatric patients are at increased risk for complications from hypothermia due to:

a) Increased body fat levels in older adults

b) Decreased ability to shiver and produce heat

c) Faster metabolic rate in older adults

d) Greater surface area of the skin

86. Wheelchair users who experience pressure ulcers frequently develop them in which areas?

a) Lower back and heels

b) Hips and shoulders

c) Elbows and knees

d) Ischial tuberosities and sacrum

87. Which medication is more likely to cause orthostatic hypotension in geriatric patients?

a) Aspirin

b) Diuretics

c) Acetaminophen

d) Antacids

88. During a lift assist call for a patient with mobility issues, which of the following should be considered to ensure a safe transfer?

a) Always rush the process to minimize discomfort

b) Use appropriate equipment such as a Hoyer lift, if available

c) Only one paramedic should handle the transfer to avoid confusion

d) The patient's wheelchair should be at least five feet away during the procedure

89. What is a potential challenge when assessing pain in patients with dementia or cognitive impairments?

a) Exaggerated pain responses

b) Inability to effectively communicate pain levels and location

c) Overuse of analgesics due to constant pain complaints

d) Heightened tolerance to pain medication

90. When considering stroke assessment, what factor may complicate recognition of stroke symptoms in patients with pre-existing disabilities?

a) Slurred speech in patients with hearing impairments

b) Numbness or weakness in limbs of patients with mobility issues

c) Confusion in patients with intellectual and developmental disabilities

d) All of the above

VIII. Airway And Ventilation Management

91. What is the most common indication for endotracheal intubation?

a) Bag-valve-mask ventilation

b) Unconscious patient with a gag reflex

c) Respiratory distress with adequate oxygen saturation

d) Inability to maintain an airway or provide adequate ventilation

92. When using pharmacological adjuncts to facilitate endotracheal intubation, which drug is most commonly used as a sedative?

a) Midazolam

b) Epinephrine

c) Paracetamol

d) Adenosine

93. Which of the following supraglottic airways is designed for blind insertion?

a) Laryngeal mask airway (LMA)

b) Endotracheal tube (ETT)

c) King LT airway

d) Nasopharyngeal airway (NPA)

94. During an endotracheal intubation, where should the tip of the tube ideally be placed?

a) At the carina

b) Above the vocal cords

c) Below the cricoid cartilage

d) In the esophagus

95. What is the primary reason for administering a paralytic agent during rapid sequence intubation (RSI)?

a) To induce sedation in the patient

b) To reduce anxiety in the patient

c) To inhibit coughing or gagging during intubation attempt

d) To increase tidal volume during positive pressure ventilation

96. Which of these supraglottic airways is appropriate for use during cardiac arrest?

a) Endotracheal tube (ETT)

b) Nasopharyngeal airway (NPA)

c) Laryngeal mask airway (LMA)

d) Oropharyngeal airway (OPA)

97. What is the primary advantage of using pharmacological adjuncts during endotracheal intubation?

a) Reduced trauma to the airway

b) Increased speed of intubation

c) Improved patient positioning

d) Easier confirmation of tube placement

98. Which choice best represents a disadvantage of supraglottic airways compared to endotracheal tubes?

a) More potential for aspiration

b) More difficult to insert

c) Limited use in pediatric patients

d) Higher chance of causing trauma to the airway

99. How can cricoid pressure be helpful during endotracheal intubation?

a) It visualizes vocal cords better

b) Reduces chances of esophageal intubation

c) Increases the chance of successful first pass intubation

d) Minimizes the risk of aspiration during intubation

100. What is the most important reason for monitoring exhaled carbon dioxide (EtCO2) after successful endotracheal intubation?

a) Confirm proper tube placement

b) Evaluate the effect of sedatives on respiratory rate

c) Measure oxygen saturation level

d) Assess lung compliance

IX. Cardiovascular Management

101. What does an ST elevation in a 12-Lead ECG potentially indicate?

a) Myocardial infarction
b) Tachycardia
c) Atrial fibrillation
d) Bradycardia

102. Which of the following rhythms would require synchronized cardioversion?

a) Ventricular tachycardia with a pulse
b) Ventricular fibrillation
c) Pulseless electrical activity (PEA)
d) Asystole

103. In a 12-Lead ECG, which leads represent the inferior wall of the heart?

a) Leads I, II, and III
b) Leads V1 and V2
c) Leads II, III, and aVF
d) Leads V5 and V6

104. What is the recommended energy setting for an initial defibrillation attempt in a patient with ventricular fibrillation or pulseless ventricular tachycardia?

a) 100 joules
b) 200 joules
c) 360 joules
d) 440 joules

105. Which of the following is NOT a recommended treatment for unstable ventricular tachycardia?

a) Synchronized cardioversion
b) Amiodarone infusion
c) CPR
d) Procainamide infusion

106. Which of the following waves represents depolarization of the ventricles in a 12-lead ECG?

a) P wave
b) QRS complex
c) T wave
d) U wave

107. What is the desired rate control target for atrial fibrillation patients without pre-excitation (Wolff-Parkinson-White)?

a) < 60 bpm
b) < 80 bpm
c) < 100 bpm
d) < 120 bpm

108. Which coronary artery is best represented by V1 and V2 leads on a 12-Lead ECG?

a) Left anterior descending artery
b) Right coronary artery
c) Left circumflex artery
d) Posterior descending artery

109. In the context of synchronized cardioversion, for an unstable patient with atrial flutter, how much energy is recommended for an initial shock?

a) 25-50 joules
b) 50-100 joules
c) 120-200 joules
d) 200-360 joules

110. What does an inverted T wave on a 12-Lead ECG potentially indicate?

a) Myocardial ischemia
b) First-degree heart block
c) Sinus arrhythmia
d) Bundle branch block

X. Pharmacology

111. Which route of medication administration provides the fastest onset of action?

a) Intravenous
b) Oral
c) Intramuscular
d) Subcutaneous

112. Which of the following typically has the least severe side effects?

a) Adrenergic medications
b) Narcotic analgesics
c) Benzodiazepines
d) Anti-inflammatory drugs

113. Contraindications for aspirin administration include:

a) Hypertension
b) Asthma
c) Stroke
d) Gastrointestinal bleeding history

114. Calculate the drug dosage for a patient needing 5 mg/kg of medication, and the patient weighs 60 kg.

a) 300 mg
b) 240 mg
c) 480 mg
d) 200 mg

115. Atropine is contraindicated in which condition?

a) Tachycardia
b) Heart block
c) Hypotension
d) Bradycardia

116. How many milliliters should be administered if a medication's concentration is 25 mg/mL, and a patient requires a dosage of 175mg?

a) 2 mL
b) 7 mL
c) 5 mL
d) 3 mL

117. Which route of medication administration is appropriate for epinephrine when emergently treating anaphylaxis?

a) Oral
b) Intravenous
c) Sublingual
d) Intramuscular

118. Lidocaine, a local anesthetic, can also be used to treat which condition?

a) hypertension
b) atrial fibrillation with rapid ventricular response (RVR)
c) acute myocardial infarction
d) congestive heart failure (CHF)

119. What is one primary contraindication for morphine administration?

a) Diabetic patients

b) Hypotension

c) Patients with a history of stroke

d) Elevated heart rate

120. Calculate the infusion rate in milliliters per hour (mL/hr) when a medication requires administration as an infusion at 3 mcg/kg/min, the medication concentration is 500 mcg/mL, and the patient weighs 80 kg.

a) 28.8 mL/hr

b) 86.4 mL/hr

c) 57.6 mL/hr

d) 43.2 mL/hr

XI. Operations

121. Which of the following is the best course of action when dealing with a hazardous materials incident?

a) Attempt to identify the hazardous material by smell

b) Enter the scene and treat injured patients immediately

c) Establish a safety perimeter and contact specialized teams

d) Mix different chemicals to try and dilute the hazardous substance

122. What does the acronym "ERG" stand for in the context of a hazardous materials incidents?

a) Emergency Response Guidebook

b) Explosive Risk Group

c) Environmental Regulations Guide

d) Equipment Replacement Guide

123. Which of the following is one of the main responsibilities of a Paramedic during a hazardous materials incident?

a) Identifying and containing the hazardous material

b) Providing overall scene management

c) Decontaminating all equipment and personnel

d) Triage, treatment, and transport of patients within their scope of practice

124. What is the purpose of establishing a "hot zone" during a hazardous materials incident?

a) To contain the area with contaminated patients

b) To designate a safe area for EMS operations/response

c) To prevent unauthorized personnel from entering the contaminated area

d) To coordinate with local law enforcement on securing the scene

125. When responding to a hazardous materials incident, what can be used to quickly identify specific information about the hazard(s) involved on scene?

a) Potential Hazards Identification Information System (PHIIS)

b) National Fire Protection Association (NFPA) 704 Diamond

c) Hazardous Materials Investigation Unit (HMIU)

d) International Fire Safety Organization (IFSO)

126. In a multiple casualty incident, what is the primary goal of triage?

a) To transport all patients immediately

b) To determine the extent of injuries for each patient

c) To stabilize and treat all patients at the scene

d) To prioritize patients based on the severity of their injuries

127. Which color-coded category of triage refers to persons who have minor injuries and can wait for treatment during a multiple casualty incident?

a) Red (Immediate)

b) Black (Deceased)

c) Yellow (Delayed)

d) Green (Minor)

128. Which of the following triage systems focuses on patient categorization during multiple casualty incidents based on respiratory rate, perfusion, and mental status?

a) START (Simple Triage and Rapid Treatment)

b) MCI (Mass Casualty Incident) System

c) SALT (Sort, Assess, Lifesaving Interventions, Treatment/Transport)

d) ABC (Airway, Breathing, Circulation) Triage

129. In a multiple casualty incident, which of the following does not affect the decision to initiate triage?

a) Resource availability

b) Number of casualties

c) Personal experience in similar situations

d) Severity and nature of injuries

130. During a mass casualty incident in which there are numerous victims with varying degrees of injury, which patients should be prioritized for immediate care and transport?

a) Patients who have suffered severe life-threatening injuries but have a high chance of survival with immediate care.

b) Patients with non-life-threatening injuries requiring basic first aid.

c) Patients who are expected to die regardless of medical interventions.

131. What is the primary goal of crime scene management at a National Registry Paramedic level?

    d) Patient's close relatives or friends working with emergency services.

    a) Gathering evidence

    b) Interrogating witnesses

    c) Ensuring scene safety and providing medical care to injured individuals

    d) Identifying suspects

132. Which of the following protective measures should a National Registry Paramedic take when responding to a crime scene?

    a) Touching all objects to establish familiarity with the scene

    b) Using a flashlight to search for hidden evidence

    c) Wearing personal protective equipment (PPE) and avoiding contaminating the scene

    d) Interviewing potential witnesses without law enforcement present

133. What should a National Registry Paramedic do if they inadvertently come across potential evidence at a crime scene?

    a) Bring it directly to law enforcement officers

    b) Place it in their pocket for safekeeping

    c) Take photographs and carefully document the finding

    d) Attempt to establish its relevance to the case

134. How should a National Registry Paramedic handle an injured suspect at a crime scene?

    a) Provide medical treatment with equal priority as any other patient on the scene

    b) Provide no medical treatment until authorized by law enforcement

    c) Call other paramedics to transport so that they are not involved in handling evidence

    d) Prioritize treatment of victims before treating the suspect

135. When coordinating with law enforcement officials at a crime scene, National Registry Paramedics should primarily focus on:

    a) Directing officers where to place barriers

    b) Taking detailed notes about officer actions and conversations

    c) Providing relevant updates on patient status and cooperating with requests to maintain scene integrity

    d) Recommending potential charges against suspects

ANSWERS

1. c) To exchange gases between the body and the environment

2. c) Pulmonary vein

3. b) Dendrite

4. b) Ball-and-socket joint

5. a) Insulin

6. b) 3

7. a) Aorta

8. c) Autonomic nervous system

10. b) Smooth muscle

11. c) Arthralgia

12. c) Difficulty breathing

13. c) Decreased oxygen in the body

14. b) A rapid heart rate

15. b) Inflammation

16. a) Release of endotoxins by bacteria

17. a) Increased preload

18. a) Massive vasodilation

19. a) Compression of the heart and great vessels, impeding venous return and cardiac output

20. c) Lack of insulin leading to the breakdown of fats for energy and increased ketone production

21. c) Ensuring scene safety

22. c) To protect the paramedic from hazards and contaminants

23. c) All individuals involved, regardless of injury severity

24. d) Media review on what happened

25. d) All the above

26. d) Past medical history

27. c) Opening the airway using head-tilt chin-lift or jaw-thrust maneuver

28. c) Pulse rate and quality

29. b) Jaw-thrust maneuver without head extension

30. d) Palpation

31. d) Height

32. b) Pneumothorax

33. a) Signs/Symptoms, Allergies, Medications, Past medical history, Last oral intake, Events leading to present illness/injury

34. d) Glucose level

35. c) Apply a cervical collar

36. b) Perform a 12-lead ECG

37. a) Epinephrine

38. c) Cardiac arrest with persistent bradycardia

39. a) Attach AED to check for shockable rhythm/arrhythmia

40. a) Chest decompression using a needle thoracostomy

41. d) Joint stiffness

42. b) Defibrillation

43. b) Albuterol

104

44. a) Smoking

45. c) Atonic seizure

46. b) Face drooping, Arm weakness, Speech difficulty, Time to call 911.

47. d) Aggressive fluid resuscitation

48. a) Type 1 diabetes

49. c) Administering a saline nebulizer treatment

50. b) Administration of supplemental oxygen.

51. a) Direct pressure

52. c) Apply direct pressure to bleeding sites

53. d) Stopping the burning process by flushing with water

54. c) Prevention of secondary injury due to movement

55. c) Full-thickness burns

56. a) Fractured extremity

57. a) Hypovolemic shock

58. b) The patient has midline neck tenderness

59. a) KED (Kendrick Extrication Device)

60. a) Percentage of body surface area affected

61. d) Evaluate their airway, breathing, and circulation (ABCs)

62. a) Appearance, work of breathing, and circulation to the skin

63. b) 30:2

64. a) This can impair venous return to the heart and reduce cerebral blood flow.

65. a) 20 mL/kg

66. d) Minimum weight-bearing ability

67. b) Back blows and chest thrusts

68. d) Adult-dose pads but with a pediatric attenuator

69. d) Amiodarone

70. c) Birth to 18 years old

71. d) Fluid-filled silicone breast implant rupture

72. b) Buttocks or feet present first

73. a) The baby's head emerges but the shoulders get stuck behind the pelvic bone

74. a) Vertex, occiput anterior

75. c) It can cause oxygen deprivation and bradycardia in the newborn if not corrected promptly

76. c) Third stage of labor

77. a) Clearing airway, ensuring there is no cord around the neck

78. b) 4

79. d) On their back with knees bent or slightly modified lithotomy position

80. a) Fundal massage

81. b) Shortened and externally rotated leg

82. b) Use written communication if possible

83. d) Emphysema

84. c) Use simple language and ask one question at a time

85. b) Decreased ability to shiver and produce heat

86. d) Ischial tuberosities and sacrum

87. b) Diuretics

88. b) Use appropriate equipment such as a Hoyer lift, if available

89. b) Inability to effectively communicate pain levels and location

90. d) All of the above

91. d) Inability to maintain an airway or provide adequate ventilation

92. a) Midazolam

93. c) King LT airway

94. b) Above the vocal cords

95. c) To inhibit coughing or gagging during intubation attempt

96. c) Laryngeal mask airway (LMA)

97. a) Reduced trauma to the airway

98. a) More potential for aspiration

99. d) Minimizes the risk of aspiration during intubation

100. a) Confirm proper tube placement

101. a) Myocardial infarction

102. a) Ventricular tachycardia with a pulse

103. c) Leads II, III, and aVF

104. b) 200 joules

105. c) CPR

106. b) QRS complex

107. c) < 100 bpm

108. a) Left anterior descending artery

109. b) 50-100 joules

110. a) Myocardial ischemia

111. a) Intravenous

112. d) Anti-inflammatory drugs

113. d) Gastrointestinal bleeding history

114. a) 300 mg

115. a) Tachycardia

116. b) 7 mL

117. d) Intramuscular

118. b) atrial fibrillation with rapid ventricular response (RVR)

119. b) Hypotension

120. b) 86.4 mL/hr

121. c) Establish a safety perimeter and contact specialized teams

122. a) Emergency Response Guidebook

123. d) Triage, treatment, and transport of patients within their scope of practice

124. c) To prevent unauthorized personnel from entering the contaminated area

125. b) National Fire Protection Association (NFPA) 704 Diamond

126. d) To prioritize patients based on the severity of their injuries

127. d) Green (Minor)

128. START (Simple Triage and Rapid Treatment)

129. c) Personal experience in similar situations

130. a) Patients who have suffered severe life-threatening injuries but have a high chance of survival with immediate care.

131. c) Ensuring scene safety and providing medical care to injured individuals

132. c) Wearing personal protective equipment (PPE) and avoiding contaminating the scene

133. c) Take photographs and carefully document the finding

134. a) Provide medical treatment with equal priority as any other patient on the scene

135. c) Providing relevant updates on patient status and cooperating with requests to maintain scene integrity

Conclusion

The journey to becoming a certified paramedic is both challenging and rewarding. The information provided in the *"National Registry Paramedic Prep"* book aims to prepare you thoroughly for the National Registry Paramedic Exam, covering a comprehensive range of topics from anatomy and cardiology to EMS operations and medical legal considerations.

As you reflect on your studies and prepare to step into this crucial role within the healthcare system, it is important to remember a few final pieces of advice. First, continue seeking out effective test-taking tips and strategies for overcoming test anxiety. Utilize study plans that incorporate time management techniques to maximize your preparation efforts.

Understanding the key concepts and skills assessed during the exam is essential, so review the material diligently. Focus on areas such as pathophysiology, medication administration, special patient populations, and trauma management as they require your keen attention.

It's crucial to practice applying your knowledge in real-life scenarios through practice exams and question-answer sessions. Active learning will help reinforce your understanding of the topics covered, ensuring that you are well-prepared when faced with emergency situations as a paramedic.

In the field of emergency medical services, every case you encounter will present unique challenges; therefore, adaptability and constant learning are essential traits for success in this profession. It is important to continually refresh your skills and stay updated on advancements in medical research and procedures.

Lastly, always be mindful of medical legal and ethical considerations while performing your duties as a paramedic. Prioritize patient care while adhering to standards of consent, documentation, and maintaining confidentiality under HIPAA regulations.

With perseverance, dedication, and unwavering commitment towards saving lives in critical situations—at times even under immense pressure—you will thrive in this rewarding career. As you embark on this journey armed with knowledge from *"National Registry Paramedic Prep,"* trust in yourself and strive for excellence. Good luck on your exam and here's to a successful future as an accredited paramedic!

Made in the USA
Monee, IL
24 November 2023

47204058R00061